Diabetic Snacks And Desserts Cookbook

By:

Maria Lancasters

TABLE OF CONTENTS

INTRODUCTION

INTRODUCTION

Diabetes is a chronic disease affecting one's ability to manage their blood sugar internally. As a result, sufferers of Diabetes are required to manage their blood sugar levels through diet, exercise, and injection of insulin. With 1.6 million new cases per year, there is a growing need for accurate diabetic diet information.

The most effective diets that diabetics can use to manage their blood sugar effectively are diets where total calories and carbohydrates are controlled. Because carbohydrates are broken down to create blood sugars, controlling the intake through specialized diets are the best way to keep blood sugar levels under control. There are several types of popular diets that can be adapted to suit the dietary requirements of a diabetic. Low-carb, high fiber, high protein diets are the most common. There are also diets that set a level of calories not to be exceeded as the more calories ingested, the more insulin that will be needed to properly metabolize the resulting sugars. Current accepted diabetic diet information dictates that any diet where carbohydrates and resulting blood sugars are controlled would be considered a viable meal plan for the management of Diabetes.

In recent years, artificial sweeteners have been developed that do not impact blood sugar levels and are thus acceptable for ingestion by diabetics. Artificial sweeteners allow diabetics to eat almost anything that a non-diabetic can consume, the only caveat being that any sugar ingredients must be replaced with an acceptable artificial sweetener such as Aspartame, Sucra, or Splenda.

The commonality amongst all of these diets is one simple fact. Processed sugars and high-carbohydrate foods have a large impact on raising blood sugar levels, requiring extensive monitoring and management through regular insulin injection. By controlling the foods that cause a rise in blood sugar levels, management (or prevention) of Diabetes becomes easier.

Clearly there is a large need for accurate diabetic diet information. Diabetes has been called a silent epidemic and informing the uninformed masses is our goal here at DiabeticDietInformation.org. Although there is promising research in the realm of Diabetes, there still is no cure. Currently, education is our best weapon against Diabetes as it is almost 100% preventable through simple lifestyle changes.

ESSENTIAL NUTRIENTS FOR A DIABETIC DIET

Diabetes is one of the most common diseases that has struck millions of people and has even taken away lives. It is alarming to find out that some people are not even aware that they have diabetes. A person can develop diabetes out of having a poor diet or could be hereditary. It can be very much avoided but if you happen to have it already, the best way to deal with the disease is by means of having a healthy and balanced diet.

There is no such thing as one diet fits all and this is the same with a diabetic diet. An ideal diet for a person with diabetes is something that fits his or her lifestyle and choice. It would be much easier to follow a diet that includes foods that you like and you are willing to try.

It may be true that if you are diabetic, you may have to avoid certain foods but it doesn't mean you can enjoy your meals anymore. A very important part of a diabetic diet is to ensure that you include the essential nutrients needed in the food. Although there are different ways of planning a diabetic diet, it is important that a diabetic understands the proportion and nutritional value of the food that is he or she is eating.

The follow nutrients should be part of a diabetic diet:

Omega-6 fatty acids

Omega-6 fatty acids actually help in fighting against diabetes neuropathy. Great sources of this crucial nutrient are in borage oil and blackcurrant oil.

Alpha-lipoic acid

The alpha-lipoic acid is an antioxidant that helps in glucose uptake. For diabetic patients that are suffering from diabetes nerve damage, alpha-lipoic acid may help.

Complex high-fiber carbs

Fiber is one of the best tools in fighting against diabetes because it is able to slow down digestion and absorption of carbs and it increases insulin sensitivity in tissues thus avoiding the rise in blood sugar levels. It is recommended that a diabetic avoids refined carbs. Excellent sources of this are oats, peas, legumes, whole grains, cereals, fruits and vegetables.

Omega 3

Omega 3 is good for the heart indeed as it protects us from the hardening of our arteries. Omega 3 is commonly found in fish oils which you can get from eating salmon, herring, mackerel and tuna.

A lot of people may be wondering why diets are a very crucial part in diabetes. Aside from the fact that having a balanced diet is beneficial, diabetes has no cure which is why the best way to manage it is by eating the right kinds of foods. If you also follow a good diabetic diet, you also lessen the risk of developing complications of diabetes such as blindness, nerve damage and other heart diseases.

1 KETO PIZZA CRUST

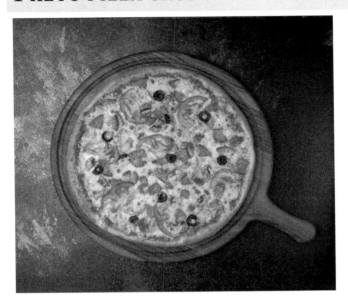

Prep Time: 8 mins

Total Time: 25 mins

Servings: 6

Ingredients

PIZZA CRUST – SPECIAL INGREDIENT
- 1 box Simple Mills Pizza Dough Almond Flour Mix

PIZZA SAUCE
- 1 Garlic Clove

- 1/2 c Heavy Whipping Cream
- 1/3 c Parmesan or Asiago Cheese (grated)
- 1/2 t Dried Oregano

TOPPINGS

- 2 oz Breakfast Sausage or Bacon
- Red Onion
- Toppings of choice

Instructions

PIZZA CRUST

• The full box produces two 8-inch crusts, so if you're making it for one person, only use half the mix. Follow the package's instructions for mixing. Spread it out to a thickness of 1/4-1/2 inch. For a total of ten minutes in the oven, bake the cookies.

PIZZA SAUCE

• Prepare your toppings and get the sauce going while the crust bakes.Thinly slice toppings (no thicker than a quarter inch) to cook rapidly.

• To warm through, place a skillet on a medium heat. Cook the sausage until it's halfway done while the pan is hot. Take out and place aside.Cook the bacon when it's crisp, then remove from heat and put aside.

• Add the garlic cloves to the oil after removing them from their skins. Anything may start stinking in a matter of seconds.

• Add the heavy cream, cheese, and oregano after that.

Reduce the heat to the lowest level as soon as the water begins to boil. As time goes on, the sauce will thicken.

ASSEMBLE THE PIZZA

• Spread the sauce on the pizza and top with the desired ingredients. Bake for another 10 minutes. OR

• If you want a perfectly crispy crust, wait until it's finished baking before adding the sauce.

• To make the crispy bacon, place it on top of the pizza once it has done baking.

Nutrition Info

1slice | Calories: 248kcal | Carbohydrates: 12g | Protein: 7g | Fat: 19g | Saturated Fat: 9g (INF%) | Polyunsaturated Fat: 0g | Monounsaturated Fat: 2g | Trans Fat: 0g | Cholesterol: 33mg (INF%) | Sodium: 268mg | Potassium: 131mg | Fiber: 2g | Sugar: 1g | Vitamin A: 400IU | Vitamin C: 8.3mg | Calcium: 140mg | Iron: 0.7mg

2 COCONUT CHIA PUDDING

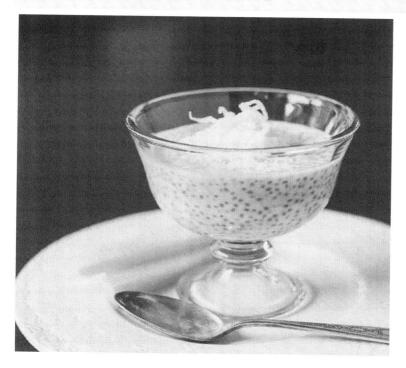

Prep Time: 15 mins
Total Time: 15 mins
Servings: 2

Ingredients

- 1/4 cups of chia seeds
- 2 tbsp shredded unsweetened coconut
- 1 & 1/4 cup light coconut milk
- 1 tsp vanilla extract
- 2 tbsp maple syrup

Instructions

- Combine all the ingredients in a large bowl.

- For 10 minutes, let it on the counter and mix it every 2-3 minutes.

- Refrigerate for 1-2 hours to firm up, covered.

- And serve

Nutrition Info

- *calories:* 235
- *sugar:* 12g
- *fat:* 10g
- *saturated fat:* 2g
- *carbohydrates:* 30g
- *fiber:* 14g
- *protein:* 6g

3 NECTARINE SLICE WITH YOGURT

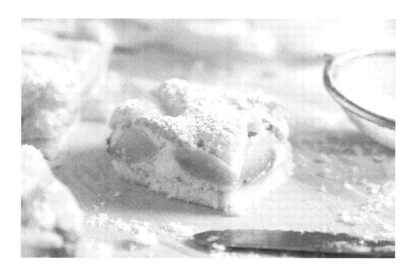

Prep Time: 10 mins
Total Time: 25 mins
Servings: 7

Ingredients

- 150g butter (without salt)
- 2 eggs (at room temperature)
- ½ cup of caster sugar
- 1 ½ cup wholemeal self-raising flour
- ¼ teaspoon bicarbonate of soda (bicarb soda)
- 1 teaspoon vanilla essence
- 1 teaspoon ground cinnamon
- 1 cup plain Greek yogurt
- ½ cup almonds, chopped
- 4 fresh nectarines, stones removed and sliced into quarters

Instructions

- Preheat oven to 180C. Line baking tray 20x30cm with baking paper
- Blend butter and sugar in a blender until white. Add in eggs one at a time
- Sift flour with bicarb and cinnamon
- Fold yogurt and flour through the egg mixture. Add in vanilla essence. Fold through ¾ fruit and all nuts gently.
- Spoon mix into the tray and flatten until smooth. Top with remaining fruit pieces.
- Bake for 20-25 minutes, or until a skewer or knife inserted into the center comes out clean. Allow 5 minutes on the tray before transferring to a cooling rack. To serve, remove the paper.

Nutrition Info

Energy- 324kJ
Protein- 2.0g
Fat - total4.5g
Fat - saturated2.0g
Carbohydrate- 7.0g
Fibre- 1.0g
Sodium -40mg

4 EASY BLACK BEAN DIP

Prep Time: 10 mins
Total Time: 10 mins
Servings: 4

Ingredients

- 1 (15 ounce) can low-sodium black beans, rinsed
- ¼ cup low-fat plain Greek yogurt
- 2 teaspoons lime juice (from 1 lime)
- ½ teaspoon ground cumin
- ½ teaspoon dried oregano
- ½ teaspoon garlic powder
- ¼ teaspoon paprika, preferably smoked
- ¼ teaspoon salt
- ¼ teaspoon ground pepper
- ¼ teaspoon cayenne pepper or ground chipotle chile (optional)
- 2 teaspoons olive oil
- ¼ cup chopped fresh cilantro or scallions
- ¼ cup chopped onion

Instructions

- Place beans, yogurt, lime juice, cumin, oregano, garlic powder, paprika, salt and pepper in a food processor or blender. Process until well combined, about 20 seconds. For a spicier dip, add cayenne (or ground chipotle) to taste, up to 1/4 teaspoon. Add oil, cilantro (or scallions) and onion. Pulse until well mixed, about 20 seconds. Transfer to a bowl to serve.

Nutrition Info

129 calories; total fat 3.4g 5%, saturated fat 0.5g; cholesterol 1mg; sodium 210mg 8%, potassium 281mg 8%, carbohydrates 17.1g

5 BERRY-MINT KEFIR SMOOTHIES

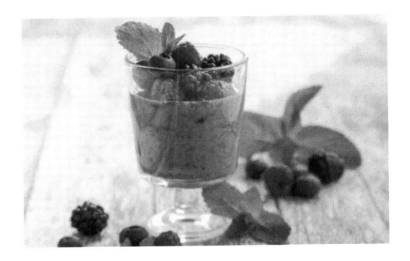

Prep Time: 5 mins
Total Time: 5 mins
Servings: 2

Ingredients

☐   1 cup low-fat plain kefir

- 1 cup frozen mixed berries
- ¼ cup orange juice
- 1-2 tablespoons fresh mint
- 1 tablespoon honey

Instructions

- Combine kefir, berries, juice, mint to taste and honey in a blender. Process until smooth. (The smoothies will keep in the refrigerator for up to 1 day or in the freezer for up to 3 months.)

Nutrition Info

137 calories; total fat 1g 2%, saturated fat 1g; cholesterol 5mg 2%, sodium 64mg 3%, potassium -1mg; carbohydrates 27g

6 LIMA BEAN HUMMUS WITH TOASTED PITA CRISPS

Prep Time: 25 mins
Total Time: 25 mins
Servings: 8

Ingredients

- 1 (10 ounce) package frozen Fordhook lima beans
- 1 (6 ounce) container plain low-fat yogurt
- 2 medium shallots, peeled and coarsely chopped (1/4 cup)
- 2 tablespoons lemon juice
- 1 tablespoon honey
- 1 tablespoon chopped fresh chives
- 2 cloves garlic
- ½ teaspoon ground black pepper
- ¼ teaspoon salt
- 3 whole-grain pita bread rounds
- Nonstick cooking spray

Instructions

- In a medium saucepan, cook lima beans in a small amount of boiling water for 10 minutes; drain.
- In a food processor, combine lima beans, yogurt, shallots, lemon juice, honey, chives, garlic, pepper and salt. Cover and process until smooth.
- Preheat oven to 400 degrees F. Halve pita bread rounds horizontally. Cut into wedges. Lightly coat pita wedges

with nonstick cooking spray. Place on a baking sheet. Bake 5 to 8 minutes or until lightly browned and crisp.
- ⬚ Serve hummus with pita crisps.

Nutrition Info

129 calories; total fat 1.1g 2%, saturated fat 0.3g; cholesterol 1mg; sodium 237mg 9%, potassium 289mg 8%, carbohydrates 25.4g

7 HONEY-BALSAMIC FRUIT SALAD

Prep Time: 10 mins
Total Time: 10 mins
Servings: 4

Ingredients

- ⬚ 1 pink or red grapefruit, peeled, sectioned, and seeded
- ⬚ 1 cup thinly sliced, cored red and/or green-skin pear
- ⬚ 2 kiwifruit, peeled and coarsely chopped
- ⬚ 3 tablespoons white or regular balsamic vinegar
- ⬚ 1 tablespoon honey

Instructions

- ⬚ Combine grapefruit sections, pear, and kiwifruit in a medium bowl.
- ⬚ Whisk together balsamic vinegar and honey in a small bowl. Pour into a sprayer. Following sprayer Instructions,

spray dressing over fruit for 10 to 15 seconds or until lightly coated, tossing fruit gently as you spray .

Nutrition Info

83 calories; total fat 0.3g 1%, saturated fatg; cholesterolmg; sodium 2mg; potassium 254mg 7%, carbohydrates 20.8g 7%, fiber 3.4g

8 PISTACHIO MUFFIN RECIPE

Prep Time: 20 mins
Total Time: 50 mins
Servings: 2

Ingredients

- nonstick cooking spray
- 1 ⅔ cups all-purpose flour
- ¾ cup white sugar
- ½ cup brown sugar
- ½ cup ground pistachio nuts
- 1 cup chopped pistachio nuts, divided
- 1 tablespoon cornstarch
- 1 teaspoon baking powder
- 1 teaspoon baking soda
- ¼ teaspoon salt
- 1 cup milk, at room temperature

- 8 tablespoons melted butter
- 2 eggs, at room temperature
- 2 teaspoons vanilla extract
- 1 teaspoon almond extract

Instructions

Step 1

Preheat the oven to 190°C (190 degrees C). Paper liners should be used to line a 12-cup muffin tray. Cooking spray the liners and the pan lightly.

Step 2

Fry butter till foamy. Add flour, brown sugar, and 1/2 cup chopped pistachios to a large mixing basin. Stir until well combined. Make a well in the middle.

Step 3

In a mixing dish, combine the milk, melted butter, eggs, vanilla extract, and almond extract. Do not overmix the milk mixture after pouring it into the dry ingredients. Stir with a spatula until just a few lumps remain after barely combining the ingredients.

Step 4

Fill muffin tins 3/4 full with the batter. The remaining pistachios should be sprinkled over the top.

Step 5

Bake for 15 minutes, or until the tops spring back when lightly pressed, flipping the pan halfway through. Allow to cool in the tin for 5 minutes. Cool completely on a wire rack.

9 ZUCCHINI PIZZA BOATS

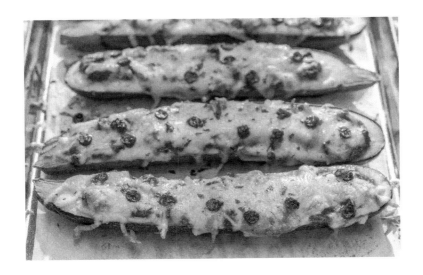

Prep Time: 15 mins
Total Time: 15 mins
Servings: 6

Ingredients

- 6 small zucchini (2 1/2 lbs)
- 1 Tbsp olive oil

- ☐ 1 clove garlic, finely minced
- ☐ Salt and freshly ground black pepper
- ☐ 1 cup marinara sauce (I used Classico Four Cheese)
- ☐ 1 1/2 cups shredded mozzarella cheese (6 oz)
- ☐ 1/3 cups finely shredded parmesan cheese (1.4 oz)
- ☐ 1/2 cup mini pepperoni slices
- ☐ 2 Tbsp chopped fresh oregano

Instructions

- Prepare the meal in the oven at 400 degrees Fahrenheit. Set a parchment paper or Silpat liner on a large rimmed baking sheet and prepare the oven.
- Cut each zucchini in half lengthwise (if the bottoms don't lay flat, remove a small amount of flesh off the bottoms to make them more flat). This was only necessary for one of them. Dry the inside completely with paper towels (cut portion). Arrange on a greased parchment paper-lined baking sheet.

- Combine the olive oil and garlic in a basin, then lightly brush the mixture over the zucchini's tops. Season with salt and pepper, then brush each zucchini with 1 tablespoon marinara sauce, leaving a rim around the sides undisturbed. Season to taste with salt and pepper.

- Top with mozzarella and then parmesan cheese, spreading the cheese evenly. Add pepperoni slices to the top to complete the look (placing them more near centers as the cheese will melt and spread). Bake for 12 to 18 minutes in a preheated oven, depending on the thickness of your zucchini and your preference for crisp/tender results.

- Remove from the oven and top with oregano leaves that have been cut finely. Ideally, serve this dish when it's still warm.

Nutrition Info

Zucchini Pizza Boats
Amount Per Serving
Calories 221Calories from Fat 126
% Daily Value*
Fat 14g
Saturated Fat 6g
Cholesterol 35mg
Sodium 660mg
Potassium 715mg
Carbohydrates 10g
Fiber 3g
Sugar 7g
Protein 13g
Vitamin A 830IU
Vitamin C 38.1mg
Calcium 273mg
Iron 2.1mg

* Percent Daily Values are based on a 2000 calorie diet.

10 CASHEW NUT COOKIES

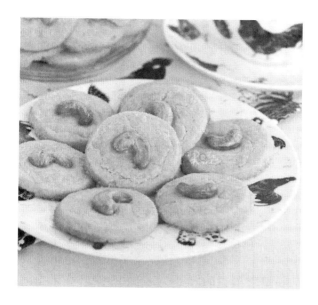

Prep Time: 20 mins
Total Time: 20 mins
Servings: 4

Ingredients

- 1/4 cup ghee or white butter
- 112 gms cashew paste
- 3/4 cup ghee
- 1 1/2 cups khaand(Muscovado)
- 20 gms flax or chia seeds
- 3 tbsp plain yogurt
- 1/2 tsp baking soda
- 1 tsp baking powder
- 1 tsp vanilla
- 1 3/4 cups oats
- 2 cups organic all-purpose flour wheat flour

Instructions

- Combine all of the ingredients(except the flour), in a large mixing basin . Now, gradually add the flour and combine all of the ingredients thoroughly to produce cookie dough.
- Refrigerate the dough for 1 hour to cool.
- Preheat oven to 160 degrees celsius and shape the dough into 1-inch round balls.
- Bake each dough ball for 10-12 minutes on an ungreased cookie sheet.
- Remove each batch from the oven and cool on a baking sheet until the cookies are completely firm.

Nutrition Info

Nuts contain unsaturated fats, protein and a range of vitamins and minerals that lower cholesterol, inflammation and insulin resistance. one should include at least 50 grams of almonds, cashews, chestnuts, walnuts or pistachios in their diet to control blood fats (triglycerides) and sugar levels. It is suggested to have 4 to 5 cashew nuts every day. You can add them to your salad, toss them in your chicken stir-fry, or add them to your sugar-free desserts.

11 VANILLA YOGURT WITH APRICOTS

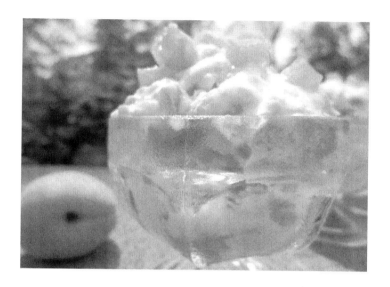

Prep Time: 5 mins
Total Time: 5 mins
Servings: 1

Ingredients

- 1 (5 ounce) container nonfat vanilla Greek yogurt
- 2 tablespoons chopped dried apricots

Instructions

- Top yogurt with apricots.

Nutrition Info

150 calories; total fat 0.3g 1%, saturated fat 0.2g; cholesterol 4mg 1%, sodium 50mg 2%, potassium 363mg 10%, carbohydrates 24.9g 8%, fiber 1.9g 8%, sugar 22g; protein 12.8g

12 SPINACH-TURKEY ROLL-UPS

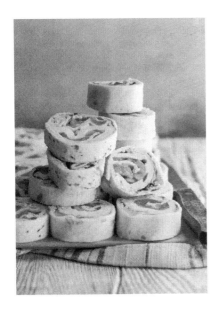

Prep Time: 20 mins
Total Time: 20 mins
Servings: 8

Ingredients

- 2 teaspoons honey mustard
- Dash ground nutmeg
- 1/2 of a (6 ounce) package thinly sliced oven-roasted or smoked turkey breast (8 thin slices)
- 1 cup fresh baby spinach leaves or fresh basil leaves
- ½ medium red or green sweet pepper, seeded and cut into thin strips
- 4 sticks low-fat string cheese, cut lengthwise into quarters
- Small fresh basil sprigs or leaves (optional)

Instructions

- In a small bowl, stir together honey mustard and nutmeg. Carefully spread mustard mixture evenly atop turkey slices. Divide the spinach (or basil leaves) among turkey slices, placing along one short edge of each turkey slice and allowing tips of leaves to extend beyond the edge of the turkey. Top with pepper strips and cheese. Starting at edge with cheese and vegetables, roll up each turkey slice. If desired, garnish turkey rolls with additional basil and cut each roll in half.

Nutrition Info

40 calories; total fat 1g 2%, saturated fat 1g; cholesterol 9mg 3%, sodium 220mg 9%, potassium -1mg; carbohydrates 2g

13 OVEN BEEF JERKY

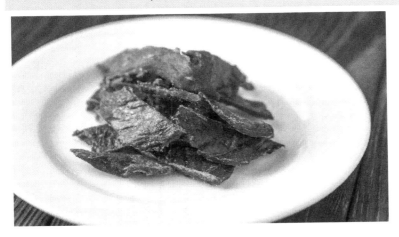

Prep Time: 20 mins
Total Time: 4hrs
Servings: 8 servings

Ingredients

- 1 pound boneless top round steak (or London broil, trimmed of fat)
- 1/4 cup liquid smoke
- 1/4 cup soy sauce
- 1/4 cup Worcestershire sauce
- 1 1/2 teaspoons kosher salt
- 1 teaspoon black pepper (freshly ground)
- 1/2 teaspoon garlic powder
- 1/2 teaspoon onion powder
- 1/2 teaspoon cayenne pepper (or to taste)

☐   1 teaspoon paprika

Instructions
- Prepare the ingredients by gathering them all at once.
- The beef should be wrapped in plastic wrap and frozen for 30 to 60 minutes, depending on how firm you want it. Cutting evenly is much simpler as a result of this.)
- Cut the meat against the grain into 1/4-inch-thick strips using a sharp knife.
- Squish the ingredients together in a big frozen bag with a zip-top closure. Add the liquid smoke after the other ingredients have been added and close the bag.

- Add the marinade and toss the meat strips to coat. Refrigerate for 12 hours or overnight after opening bag and squeezing out all the air.
- Pre-heat the oven to 250 degrees Fahrenheit. Set a jellyroll pan with a baking rack aside.
- Using paper towels, pat marinated pork strips dry.
- Place the beef strips on the jellyroll pan's baking rack in a single layer, letting air to circulate between each strip.
- Allow it bake for around four hours, or until the top feels completely dry to the touch. Wait 24 hours after you take it out of the oven for it to completely cool and dry before moving it.
- Don't let the light get to you. Retain in a container or plastic bag that can be closed tightly.

Nutrition Info

137.3 calories; protein 11.6g 23% DV; carbohydrates 4.5g 2% DV; fat 7.9g 12% DV; cholesterol 31.3mg 10% DV; sodium 934mg 37% over or resealable bags.

14 AVOCADO TURKEY LETTUCE WRAPS

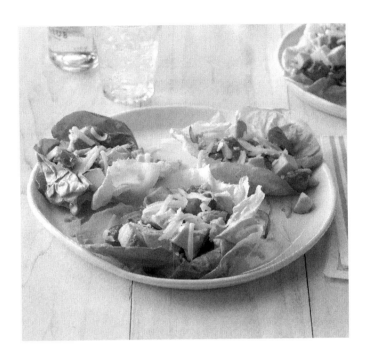

Prep Time: 10 mins
Total Time: q0 mins
Servings: 4

Ingredients

- 1 lb. Ground turkey, 93% lean
- 1 ea. Head of butterhead lettuce, leaves separated
- 2 ea. Avocados From Mexico, diced

- 1-1/2 c. Portabella mushrooms, diced
- 1-1/2 c. Brown rice, cooked
- 1 ea. Red bell pepper, diced
- 1/2 c. Onion, diced
- 1/2 c. Carrots, grated
- 2 T. Avocado oil
- 1/2 T. dried orange peel
- 4 ea. Cloves of garlic, minced
- 1/2 T. dried orange peel
- To garnish, Chives
- 1/2 t. Smoked paprika
- 1/3 c. Coconut aminos
- 1/3 c. Vegetable broth
- 1/4 c. Peanut butter
- 1 T. Rice vinegar
- 1/2 T. Ginger paste
- 1 t. Sesame oil
- Dash Chili powder
- To taste, Salt and pepper

Instructions

- Toss red pepper, onion, mushrooms, and garlic with avocado oil in a large pan over medium heat. Stirring often, cook for about 10 minutes.

- Stir in the turkey and lower the heat to medium-low. Cook the turkey for 10 to 15 minutes on each side, stirring often. After the meal has done cooking, add the carrots, orange peel, paprika, and more salt and pepper to taste.

- Before serving, mix the following ingredients in a food processor or blender: coconut aminos, vegetable broth, peanut butter, rice vinegar, ginger paste, sesame oil, and chili powder. To prepare Thai peanut sauce, puree all ingredients until smooth in a blender.

- Simmer for 5 minutes with the Thai peanut sauce after seasoning with salt and pepper.

- Garnish with chives and serve. Distribute lettuce equally on big plates. Top with brown rice.

Nutrition Info

Calories 650Total Carbohydrates 45Total Fat 41Saturated Fat 7Sugar 13

15 PB & J POPPERS

Prep Time: 15 mins
Total Time: 15 mins
Servings: 4

Ingredients

- ⅓ cup light cream cheese spread, softened
- 1 tablespoon powdered peanut butter
- ¼ teaspoon ground ginger or apple pie spice
- 12 miniature caramel corn- or apple-cinnamon-flavored rice cakes
- ¼ cup desired-flavor sugar-free preserves
- 2 tablespoons miniature semisweet chocolate pieces (optional)

Instructions

- Stir together cream cheese, peanut butter, and ginger in a small bowl. Spread evenly on rice cakes. Top evenly with preserves. If desired, sprinkle with chocolate pieces.

Nutrition Info

88 calories; total fat 3.5g 5%, saturated fat 2g; cholesterol 13mg 4%, sodium 170mg 7%, potassium 53mg

16 PEA PODS WITH DIPPING SAUCES

Prep Time: 10 mins
Total Time: 10 mins
Servings: 6

Ingredients

- 3 cups fresh pea pods or sugar snap peas
- 1 recipe Creamy Honey Mustard Sauce (see associated recipe)

Instructions

- Cook pea pods in a small amount of boiling lightly salted water in a covered medium saucepan for 2 to 4 minutes or until crisp-tender.
- Drain; cool. Chill if desired. Serve with Creamy Honey Mustard Sauce.

Nutrition Info

20 calories; total fatg; saturated fatg; cholesterolmg; sodium 10mg; potassium -1mg; carbohydrates 4g 1%, fiber 1g 4%, sugar -1g

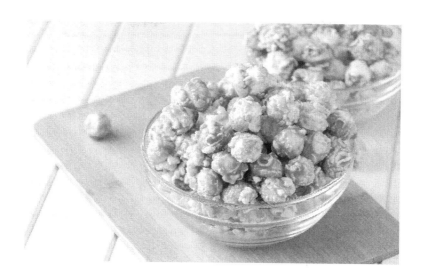

Prep Time: 5 mins
Total Time: 5 mins
Servings: 1

Ingredients

- ⬜ 1 ½ tablespoons popcorn kernels
- ⬜ 1 teaspoon olive oil
- ⬜ ½ teaspoon sesame seeds
- ⬜ ½ teaspoon poppy seeds
- ⬜ ⅛ teaspoon onion powder
- ⬜ ⅛ teaspoon garlic powder
- ⬜ Pinch of salt

Instructions

- ▢ Add popcorn kernels to a brown paper bag and fold the top of the bag over three times.
- ▢ Microwave until the popping stops, 1 to 1 1/2 minutes.
- ▢ Add oil, sesame seeds, poppy seeds, onion powder, garlic powder and salt to the bag over the popped popcorn. Fold the top of the bag, hold closed and shake to coat.

Nutrition Info

143 calories; total fat 6.8g 10%, saturated fat 0.8g; sodium 146mg 6%, potassium 25mg 1%, carbohydrates 20.8g

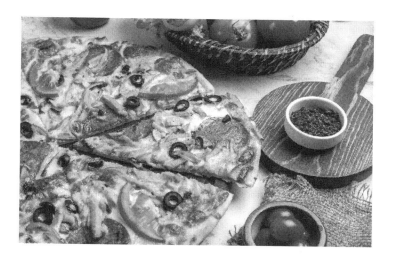

Prep Time: 15 mins
Total Time: 30 mins
Servings: 8

Ingredients

- 4 multi-grain sandwich thins, split
- ½ cup no-salt-added tomato sauce
- 1 teaspoon Italian seasoning, crushed
- ¼ teaspoon crushed red pepper
- 3 ounces thinly sliced smoked turkey sausage
- ½ cup chopped yellow or red bell pepper
- 3 ounces part skim mozzarella cheese, shredded (3/4 cup)

Instructions

- Preheat oven to 400 degrees F. Place sandwich thin halves, cut sides up, on a large baking sheet lined with parchment paper. Bake for 5 minutes.
- Meanwhile, stir together tomato sauce, Italian seasoning, and crushed red pepper in a small bowl. Spread the pre-baked sandwich thins with the sauce mixture. Top with sausage and bell pepper. Sprinkle with cheese. Bake about 8 minutes more or until the cheese is melted and bubbly. If desired, sprinkle with additional Italian seasoning.

Nutrition Info

105 calories; total fat 3.5g 5%, saturated fat 1.4g; cholesterol 14mg 5%, sodium 256mg 10%, potassium 52mg

19 FLOURLESS BANANA CHOCOLATE CHIP MINI MUFFINS

Prep Time: 20 mins
Total Time: 50 mins
Servings: 24

Ingredients

- 1 ½ cups rolled oats
- 1 teaspoon baking powder
- ¼ teaspoon baking soda
- ¼ teaspoon salt
- 2 large eggs
- 1 cup mashed ripe banana (about 2 medium-large)
- ⅓ cup packed brown sugar
- 3 tablespoons canola oil
- 1 teaspoon vanilla extract
- ½ cup mini chocolate chips

Instructions

- Preheat oven to 350 degrees F. Coat a 24-cup mini muffin tin with cooking spray.
- Pulse oats in a blender until finely ground. Add baking powder, baking soda and salt; pulse once or twice to blend. Add eggs, banana, brown sugar, oil and vanilla; puree until smooth. Stir in chocolate chips. Fill the prepared muffin cups.
- Bake until a toothpick inserted in the center comes out clean, 15 to 17 minutes. Cool in the pan on a wire rack for 5 minutes, then turn out to cool completely.

Nutrition Info

78 calories; total fat 3.6g 6%, saturated fat 0.9g; cholesterol 16mg 5%, sodium 65mg 3%, potassium 77mg

20 CHEESE SOUFFLÉ

Prep Time: 4 5 mins
Total Time: 1 hours
Servings: 5-8

Ingredients

- 300ml whole milk
- 300ml double cream
- 1 small onion, cut into quarters
- 6 cloves
- 4 fresh bay leaves
- ½ tsp lightly crushed black peppercorns
- 100g butter, plus extra for greasing
- 40g plain flour
- 750g courgettes, topped and tailed
- 1¼ tsp salt
- 225g Berkswell cheese (see tip), finely grated
- 5 large free-range eggs

Instructions

- Remove from heat and let steep for 20 minutes, then strain. Combine the milk, cream, onion, cloves, bay leaves, and peppercorns in a small saucepan.

- Return the milk to a boil and pour into a jug (discard the seasonings). In a medium-sized pan, melt 75g butter, add the flour, and cook for 1 minute, stirring constantly. Remove the remove from heat and mix in the hot milk slowly. Return the pan to the heat and cook, stirring constantly, until the sauce is silky smooth. Lower the heat and continue cooking, bring to a simmer.Meanwhile, coarsely grate the courgettes, toss them with ½ tsp of the salt and leave to drain in a colander for 10 minutes.

- Move the sauce to a large mixing bowl and set aside to cool. Squeeze out as much juice as you can from the courgettes, first by hand, then with a lot of kitchen paper or a clean tea towel. In a large frying pan, melt the remaining butter, then add the courgettes and stir-fry for 2 minutes. Remove from the equation.
- Ensure that the oven is preheated to 200 degrees Celsius (fan 180 degrees Celsius) (gas 7). 6. Lightly grease a 2.5-liter ovenproof dish (approximately 6cm deep). Shake in 25 grams of shredded cheese to cover the bottom and edges of the dish.
- Clean a big mixing basin with warm water and place the egg whites in it. Add the yolks and whisk until well-combined. Serve with 175 grams of shredded cheese, 1/4 teaspoon salt, and a generous amount of freshly ground black pepper. Stir in the courgettes. Gently fold in the egg whites once they've been whisked to stiff peaks.

- Put prepared dish on top of soufflé mixture and sprinkle with the remaining cheese. If your pie isn't golden and cooked in the center, bake it for an additional 10 minutes, then uncover and bake in the oven 10 minutes, or until it is. Serve

Nutrition Info

516kcals calories; total fat 46.5g (27.1g saturated), protein 16.4g, carbohydrates 8.5g (4.7g sugars), fibre 1.6g, salt 1.6g

21 SUPER BERRY SMOOTHIES

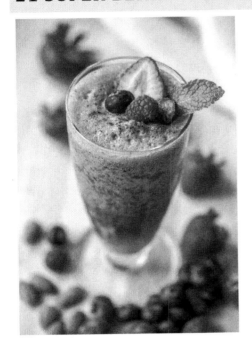

Prep Time: 10 mins
Total Time: 10 mins
Servings: 4

Ingredients

- 2 cups frozen unsweetened strawberries
- 1 cup frozen unsweetened raspberries
- 1 cup fresh blackberries or blueberries
- 1 cup fresh baby spinach leaves
- 1 cup pomegranate juice
- 3 tablespoons sugar-free vanilla-flavor protein powder, soy protein powder or nonfat dry milk powder

Instructions

- Combine strawberries, raspberries, blackberries, spinach, pomegranate juice, and protein powder in a blender. Cover and blend until smooth. Pour into glasses to serve.

Nutrition Info

118 calories; total fat 0.7g 1%, saturated fat 0.2g; cholesterol 10mg 3%, sodium 37mg 1%, potassium 325mg 9%, carbohydrates 25.7g 8%, fiber 5g 20%, sugar 17g; protein 4.6g

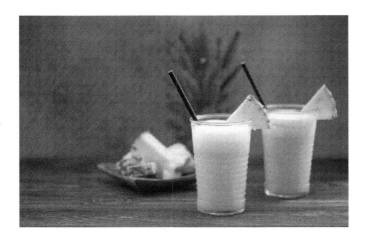

Prep Time: 10 mins
Total Time: 10 mins
Servings: 2

Ingredients

- 1 cup plain coconut water
- 1 cup frozen diced pineapple
- 1 cup packed baby spinach
- 1 small grapefruit, peeled and segmented, plus any juice squeezed from the membranes
- ½ teaspoon grated fresh ginger
- 1 cup ice

Instructions

- Combine coconut water, pineapple, spinach, grapefruit and any juices, ginger and ice in a blender. Puree until smooth and frothy.

Nutrition Info

102 calories; total fat 0.2g; saturated fatg; sodium 54mg 2%, potassium 433mg 12%, carbohydrates 25.2g 8%, fiber 2.9g

23 RICOTTA CHEESE TOAST

Prep Time: 5 mins
Total Time: 5 mins
Servings: 1

Ingredients

- ¼ cup low-fat ricotta cheese
- 3 slices whole grain toast crackers
- Freshly ground black pepper

Instructions

- Spread ricotta cheese on toasts. Sprinkle with freshly ground black pepper.

Nutrition Info

120 calories; total fat 3g; saturated fat 2g; cholesterol 20mg; sodium 150mg; potassium -1mg; carbohydrates 15g

24 CABBAGE ROLLS

Prep Time: 25 mins
Total Time: 60 hrs
Servings: 5

Ingredients

- 1 very large head of cabbage
- 1 lb. Ground turkey (white meat)
- 1/2 cup uncooked white rice
- 3/4 cup onions, diced
- 1/2 cup celery, diced
- 1 teaspoon ground white pepper
- 2 teaspoons garlic powder
- 1/2 teaspoon salt
- 2 eggs
- 1 14 1/2-oz. Can no-salt-added diced tomatoes with juice
- 1 11 1/2-oz. Bottle low-sodium V-8® juice
- Nonstick cooking spray

Instructions

- Preheat oven to 325°F.
- Coat a 9 x 13-inch glass baking dish with nonstick cooking spray. Bring a large pot of water to a gentle boil. Line a cookie sheet with paper towels.

• Take care not to rip the cabbage's broad outer leaves (you should have 10 leaves total).

- In two batches, drop the cabbage leaves into the boiling water and allow to cook for approximately 5 minutes. With a slotted spatula, remove the leaves and set them aside to cool on the baking sheet. Each leaf's tough central fiber should be removed.

- Garlic powder and salt go into a large mixing bowl with the ground turkey and the remaining ingredients. Combine thoroughly.

- To make the rolls, place about a tablespoon of the turkey mixture onto each of the cabbage leaves. Overlap the cut edges in the leaf center to keep the mixture inside, roll while folding ends toward the middle, and place in the prepared shallow dish, seam side down.

- Over the cabbage rolls, add the diced tomatoes and V-8® juice. After 40 minutes of baking, remove the foil and cook for 15–20 minutes longer, or until the sauce is bubbling. Before serving, wait the dish to cool somewhat.

Nutrition Info

Per Serving: calories: 394; carbohydrates: 51 g; total fat: 10 g; saturated fat: 3 g;

cholesterol: 156 mg; fiber: 8 g; protein: 25 g; sodium: 472 mg; carb choices: 3.5

25 PUMPKIN COCONUT ENERGY BALLS

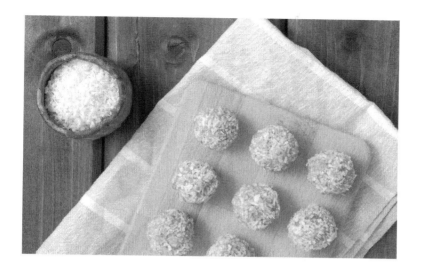

Prep Time: 20 mins
Total Time: 40 mins
Servings: 10

Ingredients

- 1 ½ cups old-fashioned oats
- ½ cup chopped slivered almonds (2 1/4 ounces)
- ⅓ cup unsweetened shredded coconut
- ¾ cup canned pumpkin
- 2 tablespoons honey
- 2 teaspoons pumpkin pie spice
- ¼ teaspoon salt
- ⅛ teaspoon cayenne pepper

Instructions

- ☐ Preheat oven to 300 degrees F.
- ☐ Place oats, almonds, and coconut on a large rimmed baking sheet. Bake, stirring once or twice, until lightly browned, 8 to 10 minutes. Cool completely on a wire rack.
- ☐ Combine pumpkin, honey, pumpkin pie spice, salt, and cayenne in a large bowl. Stir in the toasted oat mixture.
- ☐ Shape the mixture into 20 balls, about 2 teaspoons each. Place the balls on a serving tray. Serve immediately or cover and refrigerate for up to 2 days.

Nutrition Info

114 calories; total fat 5.4g 8%, saturated fat 2g; cholesterolmg; sodium 104mg 4%, potassium 127mg 4%, carbohydrates 15.2g

26 PEA PODS WITH DIPPING SAUCES

Prep Time: 10 mins
Total Time: 10 mins
Servings: 6

Ingredients

- 3 cups fresh pea pods or sugar snap peas
- 1 recipe Creamy Honey Mustard Sauce

Instructions

- Cook pea pods in a small amount of boiling lightly salted water in a covered medium saucepan for 2 to 4 minutes or until crisp-tender.
- Drain; cool. Chill if desired. Serve with Creamy Honey Mustard Sauce.

Nutrition Info

20 calories; total fatg; saturated fatg; cholesterolmg; sodium 10mg; potassium -1mg; carbohydrates 4g 1%, fiber 1g 4%, sugar -1g

27 CHUNKY ROASTED VEGGIE SPREAD

Prep Time: 25 mins
Total Time: 1 hr
Servings: 9

Ingredients

- 1 ½ pounds plum tomatoes, seeded and cut into 1-inch pieces
- 2 small red and/or yellow bell peppers, seeded and cut into 1-inch pieces
- ½ of a medium red onion, cut into 1/2-inch wedges
- 3 cloves garlic, peeled
- 2 tablespoons olive oil
- ½ teaspoon kosher salt or sea salt
- ½ teaspoon freshly ground pepper
- 2 tablespoons balsamic vinegar
- 2 teaspoons chopped fresh thyme
- ¼ cup chopped fresh basil

Instructions

- Preheat oven to 425 degrees F. Combine tomatoes, bell peppers, onion wedges, and garlic in a large bowl. Add oil, kosher salt (or sea salt), and ground pepper; toss to coat. Transfer the tomato mixture to a foil-lined shallow roasting pan.
- Roast for 35 to 40 minutes or until the vegetables are tender and slightly charred on the edges, stirring twice. Cool slightly on a wire rack.

☐ Transfer the tomato mixture to a food processor. Cover and pulse until the tomato mixture is chopped but still slightly chunky. Stir in balsamic vinegar and thyme. Stir in basil just before serving.

28 Very Veggie Smoothies

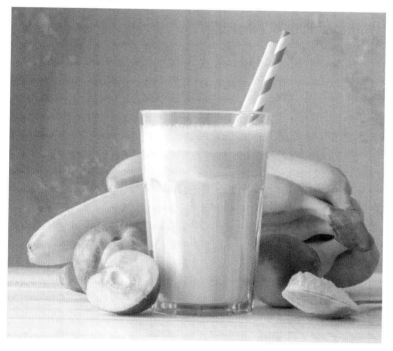

Prep Time: 10 mins
Total Time: 10 mins
Servings: 4

Ingredients

☐   2 cups ice cubes

- 2 cups V8 V-Fusion Light peach mango juice
- 1 medium peach, halved and pitted
- 1 medium banana
- 2 chard leaves, ribs removed
- Mango wedges (optional)

Instructions

- Combine ice cubes, juice, peach, banana, and chard. Cover and blend until smooth. Serve immediately. If desired, garnish with mango wedges.

Nutrition Info

68 calories; total fat 0.2g; saturated fatg; cholesterolmg; sodium 41mg 2%, potassium 292mg 8%, carbohydrates 17.2g

29 CHUNKY ROASTED VEGGIE SPREAD

Prep Time: 25 mins
Total Time: 1 hr
Servings: 9

Ingredients

- 1 ½ pounds plum tomatoes, seeded and cut into 1-inch pieces
- 2 small red and/or yellow bell peppers, seeded and cut into 1-inch pieces
- ½ of a medium red onion, cut into 1/2-inch wedges
- 3 cloves garlic, peeled
- 2 tablespoons olive oil
- ½ teaspoon kosher salt or sea salt
- ½ teaspoon freshly ground pepper
- 2 tablespoons balsamic vinegar
- 2 teaspoons chopped fresh thyme
- ¼ cup chopped fresh basil

Instructions

- Preheat oven to 425 degrees F. Combine tomatoes, bell peppers, onion wedges, and garlic in a large bowl. Add oil, kosher salt (or sea salt), and ground pepper; toss to coat. Transfer the tomato mixture to a foil-lined shallow roasting pan.
- Roast for 35 to 40 minutes or until the vegetables are tender and slightly charred on the edges, stirring twice. Cool slightly on a wire rack.

[?] Transfer the tomato mixture to a food processor. Cover and pulse until the tomato mixture is chopped but still slightly chunky. Stir in balsamic vinegar and thyme. Stir in basil just before serving.

Nutrition Info

57 calories; total fat 3.3g 5%, saturated fat 0.4g; cholesterolmg; sodium 113mg 5%, potassium 256mg 7%, carbohydrates 6.5g

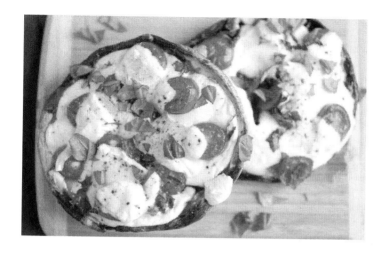

Prep Time: 10 mins
Total Time: 10 mins
Servings: 1

Ingredients

- ⬚ 1 clove minced garlic
- ⬚ 1 tbsp olive oil
- ⬚ 4 large portobello mushroom caps, cleaned
- ⬚ 1/4 tbsp salt
- ⬚ 1/8 tbsp black pepper
- ⬚ 2 tomatoes cut into 8 thin slices
- ⬚ 1 cup (4 ounces) fat shredded mozzarella cheese
- ⬚ 5 chopped basil leaves,

Instructions

- Pre-heat oven to 450F. Spray a baking sheet.

- Combine olive oil and garlic. To prepare the pan, brush the mushroom caps with the garlic mixture on all sides. Add Salt and pepper to taste flvor , then top with tomato, mozzarella, and basil.

- 7–9 minutes bake Cheese and basil on top Return to oven for 1-2 minutes to melt cheese.

Nutrition Info

Calories Per Serving: 265

35%Total Fat 22.7g

15%Cholesterol 44.2mg

15%Sodium 353.2mg

1%Total Carbohydrate 2.6g

Sugars 1.4g

26%Protein 13.1g

13%Vitamin A 117.3µg

6%Vitamin C 3.8m

31 BRUSCHETTA PLANKS

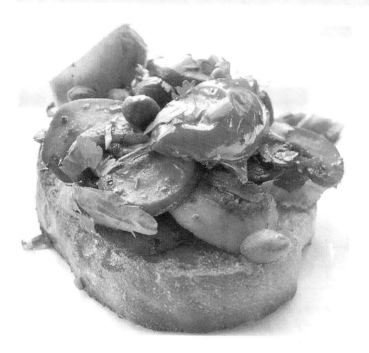

Prep Time: 10 mins
Total Time: 20 mins
Servings: 4

Ingredients

- ½ cup chopped red or yellow sweet pepper
- ½ cup chopped fresh button mushrooms or cremini mushrooms
- ¼ cup chopped onion
- 2 teaspoons olive oil

- 1 medium tomato, seeded and chopped (1/2 cup)
- 1 clove garlic, minced
- 2 tablespoons snipped fresh basil
- 4 thin whole-grain flatbread crackers
- 1 ounce Parmesan cheese, thinly shaved

Instructions

- In a medium nonstick skillet, cook sweet pepper, mushrooms and onion in hot oil over medium heat for 5 to 7 minutes or until tender, stirring occasionally. Add tomato and garlic. Cook and stir for 1 minute more. Remove from heat. Stir in basil.
- Spoon tomato mixture evenly on crackers. Top with shaved Parmesan cheese. Serve immediately.

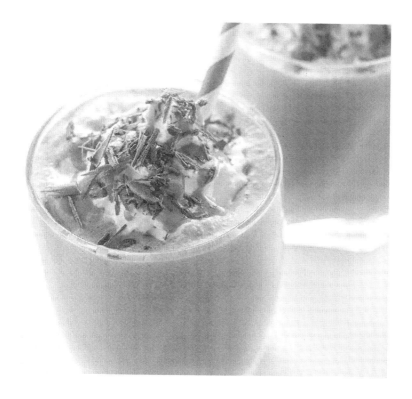

Prep Time: 5 mins
Total Time: 5 mins
Servings: 1

Ingredients

- 1/4 cup Peanut butter (creamy)
- 3 tbsp Cocoa powder
- 1 cup Heavy cream (coconut cream for dairy-free or vegan)
- 1 1/2 cup Unsweetened almond milk (regular or vanilla)
- 6 tbsp Besti Powdered Erythritol (to taste)
- 1/8 tsp Sea salt (optional)

Instructions

- Combine all ingredients in a blender.

- Puree until smooth. Adjust sweetener to taste if desired..

Nutrition Info

Amount per serving. Serving size in recipe notes above.
Calories435
Fat41g
Protein9g
Total Carbs10g
Net Carbs6g
Fiber4g
Sugar3g

33 PEPPERMINT CHECKERBOARD COOKIES

Prep Time: 40 mins
Total Time: 3 hrs 50 mins
Servings: 60

Ingredients

- ½ cup tub-style vegetable oil spread
- ½ cup sugar
- 1 teaspoon baking powder
- ¼ teaspoon salt
- 2 ounces white baking chocolate, melted and cooled slightly
- ¼ cup canola oil
- ¼ cup refrigerated or frozen egg product, thawed, or 1 egg
- 2 ½ cups flour
- ½ teaspoon peppermint extract
- Red paste food coloring

Instructions

- In a large bowl, beat vegetable oil spread, sugar, baking powder, and salt with an electric mixer on medium to high speed until well combined, scraping sides of bowl occasionally. Beat in melted white chocolate, oil, and egg. Beat in as much of the flour as you can with the mixer. Using a wooden spoon, stir in any remaining flour.
- Divide dough in half. Stir peppermint extract into one portion of dough and tint dough with red food coloring

(knead dough as needed to incorporate extract and coloring).

- Shape each portion of dough into a rectangular log that is 7 inches long and 1-1/2 inches wide. Wrap each log in plastic wrap or waxed paper. Chill logs about 2 hours or until dough is firm enough to slice. Using a long sharp knife, cut each log lengthwise into four slices. (From each color of dough, you will have four pieces that are each 7 inches long and about 1/3 inches wide.)
- Stack four pieces of dough together, alternating colors. (You will have two square logs, each with four layers.) Gently press dough together to seal layers. If necessary, wrap each log in plastic wrap or waxed paper and chill about 30 minutes or until dough is firm enough to slice.
- Cut each log lengthwise into four strips. (Each strip will have four layers in alternating colors.) Stack four strips of dough together, alternating colors, to create a checkerboard effect. Trim edges as needed to straighten sides and ends. If necessary, wrap each log in plastic wrap or waxed paper and chill about 30 minutes or until firm enough to slice.
- Preheat oven to 350 degrees F. Cut logs crosswise into 1/4-inch-thick slices. Place slices 1 inch apart on parchment paper-lined cookie sheets.
- Bake for 7 to 9 minutes or just until edges are firm. Cool on cookie sheet for 1 minute. Transfer cookies to a wire rack and let cool. To store, layer cookies between sheets of waxed paper in an airtight container. Cover and store at room temperature for up to 2 days or freeze for up to 3 months.

Nutrition Info

53 calories; total fat 2.8g 4%, saturated fat 0.5g; cholesterolmg; sodium 41mg 2%, potassium 11mg; carbohydrates 6.3g

34 POPCORN CRUNCH MIX

Prep Time: 10 mins
Total Time: 10 mins
Servings: 7

Ingredients

- 2 cups honey-nut cereal, such as Chex Honey-Nut Cereal
- 4 cups light sea-salt popcorn, such as Angie's Boom Chicka Pop Sea Salt Popcorn
- ½ cup cocoa peanuts, such as Planters Cocoa Peanuts (2 1/2 ounces)
- 1 ounce bittersweet chocolate

Instructions

- Line a large shallow pan with wax paper or parchment paper. Add honey-nut cereal, popcorn, and peanuts to pan; gently toss to combine.
- Microwave chocolate in a microwave-safe custard cup on 50% power (Medium) about 1 minute or until melted and smooth; stirring once. Drizzle over the cereal mixture. Freeze for 5 minutes. Store in an airtight container in the refrigerator for up to 2 days.

Nutrition Info

140 calories; total fat 7.2g 11%, saturated fat 1.6g; cholesterolmg; sodium 109mg 4%, potassium 104mg 3%, carbohydrates 18.1g

35 FRUITED OATMEAL COOKIES

Prep Time: 25 mins
Total Time: 35 mins
Servings: 48

Ingredients

- 2 cups rolled oats
- Nonstick cooking spray
- ½ cup butter, softened
- 1 ½ cups packed brown sugar
- ¾ teaspoon baking soda
- ¼ teaspoon salt
- ¼ teaspoon ground allspice
- 1 (6 ounce) container plain lowfat yogurt
- ½ cup refrigerated or frozen egg product, thawed, or 2 eggs, lightly beaten
- 1 teaspoon vanilla
- 2 ¼ cups flour
- ¼ cup snipped dried apricots
- ¼ cup dried currants
- ¼ cup chopped walnuts, toasted

Instructions

- Preheat oven to 375 degrees F. Spread oats in a shallow baking pan. Bake about 10 minutes or until toasted, stirring once; set aside. Lightly coat cookie sheet with cooking spray or line with parchment paper; set aside.
- In a large bowl, beat butter with an electric mixer on medium to high speed for 30 seconds. Add brown sugar,

baking soda, salt, and allspice; beat until combined. Beat in yogurt, egg and vanilla. Beat in as much of the flour as you can with the mixer. Using a wooden spoon, stir in oats, apricots, currants, walnuts, and any remaining flour. Drop dough by rounded teaspoons 2 inches apart on prepared cookie sheet.

🔲 Bake for 9 to 11 minutes or until edges and bottoms are browned. Transfer cookies to a wire rack; let cool. To store, place cookies in an airtight container; cover. Store at room temperature for up to 3 days or freeze for up to 2 months.

Nutrition Info

101 calories; total fat 2.9g 4%, saturated fat 1.4g; cholesterol 5mg 2%, sodium 55mg 2%, potassium 73mg 2%, carbohydrates 16.9g

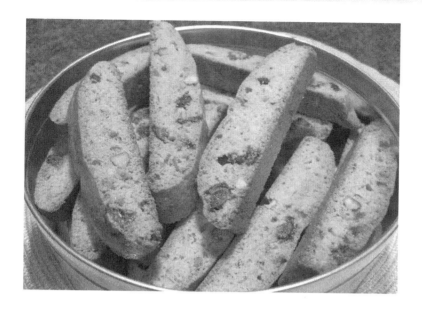

Prep Time: 30 mins
Total Time: 2 hrs 10 mins
Servings: 28

Ingredients

- Nonstick cooking spray
- ¼ cup butter, softened
- ½ cup sugar
- 1 teaspoon baking powder
- ¼ teaspoon baking soda
- ¼ teaspoon ground ginger
- ½ cup refrigerated or frozen egg product, thawed, or 2 eggs
- ½ teaspoon vanilla
- ½ cup yellow cornmeal

- 1 teaspoon finely shredded lemon peel
- 1 ⅔ cups all-purpose flour
- ⅓ cup finely chopped, stemmed dried mission figs
- 2 ounces white baking chocolate (optional)
- ½ teaspoon shortening (optional)

Instructions

- Preheat oven to 375 degrees F. Lightly coat a large cookie sheet with nonstick cooking spray; set aside. In a large mixing bowl, beat butter with an electric mixer on medium speed for 30 seconds. Add sugar, baking powder, baking soda, and ginger, beating until combined. Beat in eggs and vanilla. Beat in cornmeal and lemon peel. Beat in as much of the flour as you can with the mixer. Using a wooden spoon, stir in the remaining flour and the figs.
- Divide dough in half. Shape each portion into an 8-inch-long log. Place logs 3 inches apart on prepared cooked sheet; flatten the logs slightly until 2 inches wide. Bake for 18 to 20 minutes or until firm and a wooden toothpick inserted near center of each log comes out clean. Cool on cookie sheet on a wire rack for 1 hour.
- Preheat oven to 325 degrees F. Using a separated knife, cut each log diagonally into 1/2-inch-thick slices. Arrange slices, cut sides down, on cookie sheet. Bake 10 minutes; turn slices. Bake for 8 to 10 minutes more or until dry and crisp. Transfer to a wire rack; cool.
- If desired, in a small saucepan, heat white chocolate and shortening over very low heat until melted and smooth. Drizzle over biscotti on waxed paper; let stand until chocolate is set.

Nutrition Info

70 calories; total fat 1.8g 3%, saturated fat 1.1g; cholesterol 4mg 1%, sodium 41mg 2%, potassium 33mg 1%, carbohydrates 12.2g 4%, fiber 0.5g 2%, sugar 5g; protein 1.5g

37 HOMEMADE MULTI-SEED CRACKERS

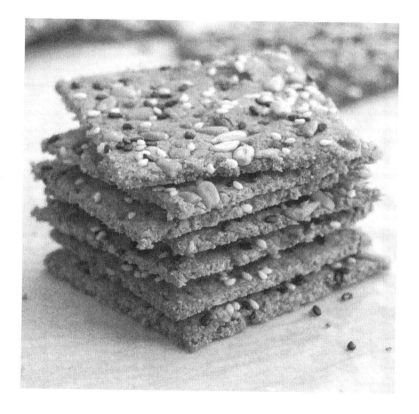

Prep Time: 25 mins
Total Time: 1 hr
Servings: 24

Ingredients

- 1 cup cooked brown rice, at room temperature
- 1 cup cooked quinoa, at room temperature
- ¼ cup sesame seeds
- ¼ cup flaxseeds
- ¼ cup sunflower seeds
- 2 tablespoons reduced-sodium tamari
- 2 tablespoons water
- ¼ teaspoon salt
- ¼ teaspoon ground pepper

Instructions

- Place oven racks in upper and lower sections of the oven. Preheat to 350 degrees F. Cut 3 pieces of parchment paper the size of a large baking sheet.
- Place rice, quinoa, sesame seeds, flaxseeds, sunflower seeds, tamari, water, salt and pepper in a food processor. Process until finely chopped and coming together in a ball. The dough will be sticky.
- Divide the dough in half. Place 1 piece of dough between 2 sheets of the prepared parchment paper. Roll out as thin as possible. Remove the top sheet of parchment and place the dough with parchment on a baking sheet. Repeat with the remaining dough and prepared parchment.
- Bake for 15 minutes. Switch the position of the baking sheets and continue baking until dark around the edges and crisp, 12 to 15 minutes more. Remove from oven and carefully break into roughly shaped crackers. If some

crackers aren't fully crisp, return them to the oven and bake for 5 to 10 minutes more.

Nutrition Info

47 calories; total fat 2.5g 4%, saturated fat 0.3g; sodium 84mg 3%, potassium 49mg 1%, carbohydrates 5g 2%, fiber 1.2g 5%, sugarg; protein 1.6g

38 PUMPKIN COCONUT ENERGY BALLS

Prep Time: 20 mins
Total Time: 40 mins
Servings: 10

Ingredients

- 1 ½ cups old-fashioned oats
- ½ cup chopped slivered almonds (2 1/4 ounces)
- ⅓ cup unsweetened shredded coconut
- ¾ cup canned pumpkin
- 2 tablespoons honey
- 2 teaspoons pumpkin pie spice
- ¼ teaspoon salt
- ⅛ teaspoon cayenne pepper

Instructions

- Preheat oven to 300 degrees F.

- Place oats, almonds, and coconut on a large rimmed baking sheet. Bake, stirring once or twice, until lightly browned, 8 to 10 minutes. Cool completely on a wire rack.
- Combine pumpkin, honey, pumpkin pie spice, salt, and cayenne in a large bowl. Stir in the toasted oat mixture.
- Shape the mixture into 20 balls, about 2 teaspoons each. Place the balls on a serving tray. Serve immediately or cover and refrigerate for up to 2 days.

Nutrition Info

114 calories; total fat 5.4g 8%, saturated fat 2g; cholesterolmg; sodium 104mg 4%, potassium 127mg 4%, carbohydrates 15.2g

39 VEG-OUT CAR SNACK

Prep Time: 15 mins
Total Time: 15 mins
Servings: 7

Ingredients

- 1 cup baby carrots
- 2 cups fresh sugar snap pea pods
- 2 cups jicama, cut into sticks
- 1 cup grape tomatoes
- 1 red bell pepper, cut into strips

Instructions

- Combine the carrots, sugar snap peas, jicama sticks, tomatoes and bell pepper strips in a large bowl.
- Transfer veggie mixture to a large resealable bag or divide to fill 7 pint-sized resealable bags. Keep cold in a portable cooler.

Nutrition Info

41 calories; total fat 0.2g; saturated fatg; cholesterolmg; sodium 22mg 1%, potassium 206mg 6%, carbohydrates 8.8g

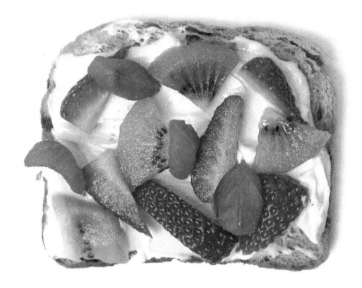

Prep Time: 5 mins
Total Time: 5 mins
Servings: 1

Ingredients

- 2 tablespoons nonfat strawberry Greek yogurt
- 1 tablespoon cream cheese
- 1 slice 100% whole-wheat bread, toasted
- ½ kiwifruit, peeled and sliced
- 1 strawberry, stems removed and sliced

Instructions

- ⬜ Combine yogurt and cream cheese in a small bowl.
- ⬜ Spread the yogurt mixture on toast and top with kiwi and strawberry.

Nutrition Info

187 calories; total fat 6.3g 10%, saturated fat 3.2g; cholesterol 16mg 5%, sodium 202mg 8%, potassium 283mg 8%, carbohydrates 24.7g

41 HONEY-BALSAMIC FRUIT SALAD

Prep Time: 10 mins
Total Time: 10 mins
Servings: 4

Ingredients

- 1 pink or red grapefruit, peeled, sectioned, and seeded
- 1 cup thinly sliced, cored red and/or green-skin pear
- 2 kiwifruit, peeled and coarsely chopped
- 3 tablespoons white or regular balsamic vinegar
- 1 tablespoon honey

Instructions

- Combine grapefruit sections, pear, and kiwifruit in a medium bowl.
- Whisk together balsamic vinegar and honey in a small bowl. Pour into a sprayer. Following sprayer Instructions, spray dressing over fruit for 10 to 15 seconds or until lightly coated, tossing fruit gently as you spray .

Nutrition Info

83 calories; total fat 0.3g 1%, saturated fatg; cholesterolmg; sodium 2mg; potassium 254mg 7%, carbohydrates 20.8g

42 CRAN-WALNUT KETTLE CORN

Prep Time: 10 mins
Total Time: 10 mins
Servings: 8

Ingredients

- 8 cups popped 94%-fat-free microwave kettle corn
- ¾ teaspoon ground cinnamon
- ½ cup dried cranberries
- ½ cup walnut pieces, toasted

Instructions

- Place popcorn in a gallon size resealable bag. To ensure even coverage, sprinkle half the cinnamon over the popcorn and shake to coat. Repeat.
- Add cranberries and walnuts to the bag; shake to combine.

Nutrition Info

97 calories; total fat 5.4g 8%, saturated fat 0.5g; cholesterolmg; sodium 50mg 2%, potassium 36mg 1%, carbohydrates 13.4g

43 ORANGE-ALMOND SLICES

Prep Time: 25 mins
Total Time: 2 hrs
Servings: 40

Ingredients

- ¾ cup sugar
- ½ cup butter, softened
- 2 eggs
- 5 ½ cups all-purpose flour
- 1 teaspoon baking powder
- ½ teaspoon salt
- ⅓ cup slivered almonds, toasted and chopped
- 1 tablespoon finely shredded orange peel

Instructions

- Preheat oven to 350 degrees F. In large bowl, combine sugar, butter and eggs. Beat with electric mixer on low to medium speed until combined. Beat in 2 cups of the flour, the baking powder, and salt. Stir in remaining flour, the almonds, and orange peel.
- Divide dough in half. Shape each half into 10-inch roll. Place on ungreased cookie sheet; flatten slightly until about 3 inches wide. Bake about 20 minutes or until toothpick inserted near center comes out clean. Cool on cookie sheet for 30 minutes.
- Preheat oven to 350 degrees F. Cut each roll into 1/2-inch slices. Place, cut sides down, on ungreased cookie sheet. Bake for 8 minutes. Turn slices over and bake for 7 to 9

minutes more or until golden and crisp. Transfer to wire rack; cool.

44 PEAR & COTTAGE CHEESE

Prep Time: 5 mins
Total Time: 5 mins
Servings: 1

Ingredients

- ¼ cup low-fat cottage cheese
- 1 tablespoon pepitas
- 1 medium pear, sliced

Instructions

- Top cottage cheese with pepitas. Serve with pear slices.

Nutrition Info

160 calories; total fat 1.6g 2%, saturated fat 0.5g; cholesterol 2mg 1%, sodium 232mg 9%, potassium 292mg

45 FAUX BAKLAVA

Prep Time: 25 mins
Total Time: 35 mins
Servings: 12

Ingredients

- ½ (17.25 ounce) package (1 sheet) frozen puff pastry
- ¾ cup sliced or slivered almonds
- 5 tablespoons honey
- ¼ teaspoon vanilla extract
- ¼ teaspoon ground cinnamon

Instructions

- Thaw puff pastry according to package Instructions. Preheat oven to 400 degrees F. Line a baking sheet with parchment paper. Using a pizza cutter, cut pastry into six pieces (each about 5 inches long and 3 inches wide). Place pastry pieces on prepared baking sheet. Bake for 10 to 12 minutes or until golden. Using a wide metal spatula, transfer pastry pieces to a wire rack.
- Meanwhile, place almonds in a large skillet; cook over medium heat about 8 minutes or until lightly browned, stirring frequently. Set aside 2 tablespoons of the almonds. In a small food processor, combine the remaining almonds, 3 tablespoons of the honey, the vanilla, and cinnamon; cover and process until ground into a thick mixture.
- Gently split each slightly warm pastry piece horizontally into two layers. Carefully spoon almond mixture in small

dollops on bottoms of pastry layers. Replace top layers of pastry. Using a pizza cutter, cut each pastry in half crosswise and then cut diagonally in half, to make four triangles per pastry.

☐ Spoon the remaining 2 tablespoons honey into a glass measuring cup. Microwave on 100 percent power (high) about 10 seconds or until thinned and a pourable consistency. Drizzle the warm honey over the pastry triangles. Sprinkle with the reserved 2 tablespoons toasted almonds.

Nutrition Info

173 calories; total fat 10.6g 16%, saturated fat 2.2g; cholesterolmg; sodium 51mg 2%, potassium 58mg 2%, carbohydrates 17.7g

Prep Time: 5 mins
Total Time: 25 mins
Servings: 4

Ingredients

PREP
- 6 tablespoons Unsalted Butter (softened)
- 4 each Large Eggs
- 1 teaspoon Vanilla Extract
- 1 tablespoon Lemon Juice (fresh)

MASH & MIX
- 2 each Medium Bananas
- ¼ teaspoon Salt (omit if using salted butter)
- 1/3 cup Coconut Flour
- 1 cup Blueberries

Instructions

PREP
- Preheat the oven to 375°.
- If the butter hasn't been softened yet, microwave it for 15 seconds in a big mixing basin.
- Beat the eggs, vanilla, and lemon juice in a small bowl for 10 seconds.

MASH & MIX
- With a fork, mash and combine the butter and bananas in a medium bowl. Chunks are OK.

- Add the egg mixture to the butter and bananas and mix well. Chunks are okay.
- Add the coconut flour and salt and mix well. The batter will be thick and possibly lumpy.
- Add the blueberries and gently mix them in without popping them.
- BAKE
- Scoop 2 tablespoons for each cookie and place on the baking sheet. Bake for 13 minutes, until the top middle is done. NOTE – cookies will not change in appearance. You need to touch the tops of a few to see if they're firm.

Nutrition Info

3cookies | Calories: 227kcal (10%) | Carbohydrates: 16g (11%) | Protein: 6g (4%) | Fat: 16g (12%) | Monounsaturated Fat: 3g | Trans Fat: 0.5g (500%) | Sodium: 161mg (11%) | Potassium: 245mg (5%) | Fiber: 4g (10%) | Sugar: 8g (9%) | Vitamin A: 593IU (3%) | Vitamin B2: 0.2mg (6%) | Vitamin B3: 0.4mg (1%) | Vitamin B6: 0.2mg (7%) | Vitamin B12: 0.3µg (1%) | Vitamin C: 7mg (4%) | Vitamin D: 82µg (456%) | Vitamin E: 0.5mg (3%) | Vitamin K: 6µg (6%) | Calcium: 21mg (1%) | Copper: 0.1mg (2%) | Folate: 27µg (4%) | Iron: 1mg (5%) | Magnesium: 18mg (4%) | Selenium: 2µg (2%) | Zinc: 0.2mg (1%) | Choline: 9.4mg (1%) | Omega-3: 0.1g (3%) | Omega-6: 0.3g (23%) | Retinol: 95ug (4%)

47 PARMESAN CARROT CRISPS

Prep Time: 15 mins
Total Time: 1 hr
Servings: 18

Ingredients

- 1 ½ cups whole-wheat pastry flour
- 1 cup finely shredded Parmesan or Gruyère cheese
- ¾ cup finely shredded carrot
- 2 tablespoons chopped fresh thyme or 2 teaspoons dried
- 1 teaspoon baking powder
- ¼ teaspoon salt
- ⅓ cup cold butter, diced
- ¼ cup water
- ⅛ teaspoon ground pepper
- Apricot fruit spread or fig preserves (optional)

Instructions

- Preheat oven to 325 degrees F.
- Combine flour, cheese, carrot, thyme, baking powder and salt in a large bowl. Stir with a fork until well combined. Using a pastry blender, cut in butter until the mixture resembles coarse crumbs and starts to stick together. Add water and stir with the fork just until combined. Gather the dough into a ball and shape into a square.
- Place the dough between sheets of parchment paper and roll out to a 10x10-inch square about 1/8-inch thick. (If necessary, remove the top sheet and use your hands to

reshape the dough into a s□uare.) Transfer to a baking sheet. Cut the dough into 18 long rectangles about 1x5 inches each . Separate the rectangles and sprinkle them lightly with pepper.

☐   Bake the crisps until the centers are firm to the touch and edges are evenly browned, 40 to 50 minutes. Cool on the pan on a wire rack for about 5 minutes. Separate the crisps and transfer to the rack to cool completely.

☐   Serve with fruit spread (or preserves), if desired. Store in an airtight container or sealable bag for up to 24 hours.

Nutrition Info

109 calories; total fat 5g 8%, saturated fat 3g; cholesterol 12mg 4%, sodium 139mg 6%, potassium -1mg; carbohydrates 13g

48 HINT-OF-HERB BUTTER COOKIES

Prep Time: 20 mins
Total Time: 4 hrs 35 mins
Servings: 48

Ingredients

- ½ cup butter
- 1 cup sugar
- 1 egg
- 1 ½ cups all-purpose flour
- 1 teaspoon baking powder
- ¼ teaspoon salt
- Fresh lavender, tarragon, lemon verbena, mint, thyme and/or herb seeds (such as anise, fennel, sesame, or poppy)

Instructions

- In a medium bowl, beat butter with an electric mixer on medium to high speed for 30 seconds. Add sugar; beat until combined. Add egg; beat until combined. Beat in flour, baking powder and salt. Divide dough in half.
- Shape each half of the dough into a 12-inch-long rope. Wrap and freeze about 4 hours or until firm.
- Preheat oven to 325 degrees F. Unwrap dough; carefully slice the frozen dough into 1/2-inch-thick slices. Place the slices, cut sides up, on a parchment paper-lined cookie sheet. Top with desired herb or seeds; press in gently, if necessary.

- ☐ Bake for 12 to 15 minutes or until edges are golden brown. Remove from cookie sheets; cool on a wire rack.

Nutrition Info

48 calories; total fat 2g 3%, saturated fat 1g; cholesterol 10mg 3%, sodium 33mg 1%, potassium -1mg; carbohydrates 7g

49 PISTACHIO & PEACH TOAST

Prep Time: 5 mins
Total Time: 5 mins
Servings: 1

Ingredients

- 1 tablespoon part-skim ricotta cheese
- 1 teaspoon honey, divided
- ⅛ teaspoon cinnamon
- 1 slice 100% whole-wheat bread, toasted
- ½ medium peach, sliced
- 1 tablespoon chopped pistachios

Instructions

- Combine ricotta, ½ teaspoon honey and cinnamon in a small bowl.
- Spread the ricotta mixture on toast and top with peach and pistachios. Drizzle with the remaining 1/2 teaspoon honey.

Nutrition Info

193 calories; total fat 6g 9%, saturated fat 1.4g; cholesterol 5mg 2%, sodium 157mg 6%, potassium 326mg

50 LEMON-PEPPER CUCUMBERS

Prep Time: 5 mins
Total Time: 5 mins
Servings: 1

Ingredients

- ½ large cucumbers, sliced (see Tip)
- Lemon juice
- Ground black pepper

Instructions

- Drizzle freshly squeezed lemon juice and freshly ground black pepper over the cucumber slices.

Nutrition Info

24 calories; total fat 0.2g; saturated fat 0.1g; cholesterolmg; sodium 3mg; potassium 230mg; carbohydrates 6g

51 OAT-WALNUT GRANOLA AND YOGURT

Prep Time: 15 mins
Total Time: 45 mins
Servings: 10

Ingredients

- Nonstick cooking spray
- 2 cups regular rolled oats
- 1 cup bran cereal flakes
- ¾ cup puffed kamut cereal or puffed wheat cereal
- ⅓ cup chopped walnuts
- ⅓ cup sugar-free or light pancake syrup
- 2 tablespoons canola oil
- ½ teaspoon ground cinnamon
- ⅛ teaspoon salt
- 5 cups plain low-fat yogurt

Instructions

- Preheat oven to 325 degrees F. Lightly coat a 15x10x1-inch baking pan with cooking spray; set aside. In a large bowl, stir together oats, bran flakes, puffed kamut cereal, and walnuts. In a small bowl, combine syrup, oil, cinnamon, and salt. Pour over oat mixture, tossing just until coated.
- Spread oat mixture evenly in prepared pan. Bake, uncovered, for 30 to 35 minutes or until oats are lightly browned, stirring twice. Remove from oven. Immediately turn out onto a large piece of foil and cool completely.

- For each serving, spoon 1/2 cup yogurt into a dish. Top with 1/3 cup granola. To store granola, place it in an airtight container and store at room temperature for up to 2 weeks.

Nutrition Info

269 calories; total fat 9.4g 14%, saturated fat 2g; cholesterol 7mg 2%, sodium 157mg 6%, potassium 466mg

52 CINNAMON-SUGAR ROASTED CHICKPEAS

Prep Time: 5 mins
Total Time: 55 mins
Servings: 4

Ingredients

- 1 (15 ounce) can chickpeas, rinsed
- 1 tablespoon sugar
- 1 teaspoon ground cinnamon
- ⅛ teaspoon ground pepper
- 1 tablespoon avocado oil

Instructions

- Position rack in the upper third of oven; preheat to 450 degrees F.
- Blot chickpeas dry. Spread on a rimmed baking sheet. Bake for 10 minutes. Meanwhile mix sugar, cinnamon and pepper in a small bowl.

▢ Transfer the chickpeas to a medium bowl and toss with oil and the cinnamon-sugar mixture. Return to the baking sheet and bake, stirring once, until browned and crunchy, 15 to 20 minutes more. Let cool on the baking sheet for 15 minutes.

Nutrition Info

125 calories; total fat 4.5g 7%, saturated fat 0.4g; sodium 48mg 2%, potassium 190mg 5%, carbohydrates 16.4g

53 CRANBERRY-ALMOND BREAD

Prep Time: 25 mins
Total Time: 1 hr 25 mins
Servings: 12

Ingredients

- 1 ½ cups whole wheat pastry flour
- ½ cup all-purpose flour
- ½ cup granulated sugar
- 1 tablespoon baking powder
- ¼ teaspoon salt
- ⅓ cup almond paste
- ¼ cup refrigerated or frozen egg product, thawed, or 1 egg, lightly beaten
- 3 tablespoons canola oil
- 1 cup fat-free milk
- ⅔ cup fresh cranberries, chopped
- ⅓ cup chopped almonds, toasted
- 2 teaspoons powdered sugar

Instructions

- Preheat oven to 350 degrees F. Grease the bottom and 1/2 inch up the sides of an 8x4x2-inch loaf pan; set aside. In a large bowl, stir together whole wheat flour, all-purpose flour, sugar, baking powder, and salt. Make a well in the center of the flour mixture; set aside.
- In a medium bowl, stir together almond paste, egg, and oil until smooth. Stir in milk. Add milk mixture all at once to flour mixture; stir just until moistened (batter should be

lumpy). Fold in cranberries and almonds. Spoon batter into prepared loaf pan.

⬚ Bake for 50 to 55 minutes or until a toothpick inserted near the center comes out clean. Cool in pan on a wire rack for 10 minutes. Remove from pan. Cool completely on wire rack. Wrap and store overnight before slicing. Sprinkle lightly with powdered sugar before serving.

Nutrition Info

177 calories; total fat 6.7g 10%, saturated fat 0.5g; cholesterolmg; sodium 158mg 6%, potassium 131mg 4%, carbohydrates 26.7g

54 KRINGLA

Prep Time: 45 mins
Total Time: 4 hrs 50 mins
Servings: 36

Ingredients

- ¾ cup sugar
- ½ cup cooking oil
- ¾ cup buttermilk
- 2 egg yolks
- 1 tablespoon vanilla
- ½ teaspoon baking soda
- 3 cups all-purpose flour
- 1 teaspoon baking powder
- Powdered sugar

Instructions

- In a large bowl, stir together sugar and oil. Add 1/2 cup of the buttermilk, the egg yolks, and vanilla. Whisk until batter is smooth. Add the remaining 1/4 cup buttermilk and the baking soda; stir just until combined. Stir together 1 cup of the flour and the baking powder; add to buttermilk mixture. Whisk until smooth. Gradually add the remaining flour, stirring until well mixed. Cover and chill dough for 4 to 24 hours.
- Preheat oven to 450 degrees F. On a lightly floured surface, drop 1 rounded tablespoon of the dough; roll into a 9- to 10-inch-long rope. About 1 inch from ends, cross one end of the rope over the other end of the rope to form

an oval. Lift ends across to opposite side of circle; press to seal. Repeat with remaining dough. Place cookies about 1 inch apart on ungreased cookie sheet lined with parchment paper.

▢ Bake about 6 minutes or just until starting to brown. Remove from cookie sheet and place on a clean kitchen towel; cover with another clean kitchen towel. Cool completely. To serve, sprinkle tops of cookies with powdered sugar.

Nutrition Info

86 calories; total fat 3.4g 5%, saturated fat 0.6g; cholesterol 12mg 4%, sodium 30mg 1%, potassium 21mg 1%, carbohydrates 12.3g

55 DOUBLE APRICOT BREAD

Prep Time: 20 mins
Total Time: 2 hrs 15 mins
Servings: 18

Ingredients

- 1 16-ounce can apricot halves, drained
- 1 ¾ cups all-purpose flour
- ¾ cup whole-wheat flour
- 1 ¼ cups sugar
- 3 ½ teaspoons baking powder
- 1 teaspoon salt
- ½ teaspoon pumpkin pie spice
- 2 eggs, beaten
- ½ cup milk
- 3 tablespoons cooking oil
- 1 cup snipped dried apricots

Instructions

- In a blender container or food processor bowl blend or process canned apricot halves until smooth. Set apricot puree aside.
- In a large bowl combine all-purpose flour, whole-wheat flour, sugar, baking powder, salt and pumpkin pie spice. In another bowl combine eggs, the apricot puree, milk and cooking oil. Add to flour mixture, stirring just until combined. Stir in snipped dried apricots. Pour into two greased and floured 8x4x2-inch or 7 1/2x3 1/2x2-inch loaf pan with bottom lined with parchment paper.

▢ Bake in a 350 degree F oven 45 to 50 minutes or until a toothpick inserted near center comes out clean. Cool in pans 10 minutes. Remove from pans. Cool completely; remove parchment paper. Slice and serve with margarine or butter, if desired.

Nutrition Info

132 calories; total fat 3g 5%, saturated fat 0.6g; cholesterol 18mg 6%, sodium 165mg 7%, potassium 138mg 4%, carbohydrates 24.9g

56 STUFFED MUSHROOMS

Prep Time: 20 mins
Total Time: 25 mins
Servings: 12

Ingredients

- 24 fresh mushrooms, 1-1/2 to 2 inches in diameter
- Nonstick cooking spray
- ¾ cup light dairy sour cream
- ½ cup finely shredded carrot
- ½ cup finely chopped red or yellow sweet pepper
- 1 green onion, finely chopped
- 1 clove garlic, minced
- Dash salt
- Dash black pepper
- 24 very tiny broccoli florets
- Black pepper (optional)

Instructions

- Preheat oven to 425 degrees F. Line a 15x10x1-inch baking pan with foil. Remove stems from mushrooms and discard or save for another use. Place mushroom caps, stem sides down, in prepared pan. Lightly coat the rounded side of each mushroom cap with nonstick cooking spray. Bake about 5 minutes or just until tender. Carefully place mushroom caps, stem sides down, on a double thickness of paper towels to cool.
- Meanwhile, in a small bowl, combine sour cream, carrot, sweet pepper, green onion, garlic, salt, and the dash black

pepper. Place cooled mushroom caps, stem sides up, on a platter. Spoon a scant tablespoon of the sour cream mixture into each mushroom cap. Top each with a broccoli floret. If desired, sprinkle with additional black pepper. Serve immediately.

Nutrition Info

29 calories; total fat 1.4g 2%, saturated fat 0.8g; cholesterol 4mg 1%, sodium 26mg 1%, potassium 178mg 5%, carbohydrates 3.2g

57 TAHINI-YOGURT DIP

Prep Time: 10 mins
Total Time: 10 mins
Servings: 4

Ingredients

- 2 tablespoons tahini
- 1 tablespoon lemon juice, plus more to taste
- 1 clove garlic, minced
- ¼ teaspoon salt
- 1 cup low-fat plain Greek yogurt
- ¼ cup chopped fresh cilantro

Instructions

- Combine tahini, lemon juice, garlic and salt in a small bowl and mix until smooth. Mix in yogurt and cilantro and stir well to combine. Add more lemon juice, if desired. Transfer to a bowl to serve.

Nutrition Info

88 calories; total fat 5.1g 8%, saturated fat 1.3g; cholesterol 6mg 2%, sodium 168mg 7%, potassium 127mg 4%, carbohydrates 4.4g

58 JAVA CUPCAKES

Prep Time: 30 mins
Total Time: 45 mins
Servings: 8

Ingredients

- 2 ½ cups sifted cake flour or 2 1/4 cups all-purpose flour
- ⅓ cup unsweetened cocoa powder
- 2 tablespoons instant espresso coffee powder or instant coffee crystals
- 1 ½ teaspoons baking powder
- ½ teaspoon baking soda
- ¼ teaspoon salt
- 1 ¼ cups buttermilk or sour fat-free milk
- 1 ¼ cups granulated sugar
- ½ cup canola oil or cooking oil
- ½ cup refrigerated or frozen egg product, thawed, or 2 eggs
- 2 teaspoons vanilla
- 1 teaspoon powdered sugar and/or unsweetened cocoa powder

Instructions

- Preheat oven to 350 degrees F. Line twenty-one 2 1/2-inch muffin cups with paper bake cups or coat with nonstick cooking spray; set aside. In a large bowl, combine flour, cocoa powder, espresso powder, baking powder, baking soda and salt.

- In another large bowl, whisk together buttermilk, granulated sugar, oil, eggs and vanilla. Add buttermilk mixture to flour mixture. Beat mixture with a wire whisk just until combined.
- Fill muffin cups 2/3 full with batter. Bake about 15 minutes or until tops spring back when lightly touched. Cool in cups on a wire rack 5 minutes. Remove from cups.
- Cool completely. Sprinkle with powdered sugar and/or cocoa powder.

Nutrition Info

169 calories; total fat 5.6g 9%, saturated fat 0.5g; cholesterol 1mg; sodium 102mg 4%, potassium 66mg 2%, carbohydrates 26.5g

59 TANGERINE BISCOTTI

Prep Time: 25 mins
Total Time: 4 hrs
Servings: 32

Ingredients

- 1 ½ cups all-purpose flour
- ½ cup whole wheat flour
- 2 teaspoons baking powder
- 2 tablespoons finely shredded tangerine peel or orange peel
- ¼ cup butter (no substitutes)
- ½ cup sugar
- ½ cup refrigerated or frozen egg substitute, thawed, or 2 eggs
- 1 teaspoon vanilla

Instructions

- Stir together all-purpose flour, whole wheat flour, baking powder, and tangerine peel in a medium mixing bowl. Set aside. Beat butter in a large mixing bowl with an electric mixer on medium speed for 30 seconds. Add sugar; beat until combined. Add egg substitute and vanilla; beat well. Stir in flour mixture.
- Preheat oven to 375 degrees F. Shape dough into two 12-inch-long logs. Place logs on a cookie sheet; flatten logs slightly until about 1-3/4 inches wide.
- Bake for 15 to 20 minutes or until lightly browned. Cool completely on cookie sheet (about 1 hour).

☐ Reheat oven to 325 degrees F. Cut each log diagonally into 1/2-inch-thick slices. Arrange the slices, cut sides down, on the cookie sheet. Bake for 10 minutes. Turn over. Bake for 10 to 12 minutes more or until crisp and light brown. Transfer to wire racks and cool completely.

Nutrition Info

55 calories; total fat 1.5g 2%, saturated fat 0.9g; cholesterol 4mg 1%, sodium 33mg 1%, potassium 21mg 1%, carbohydrates 9g

60 TURKEY VEGETABLE ROLL-UPS

Prep Time: 20 mins
Total Time: 1 hr 20 mins
Servings: 8

Ingredients

- 8 slices deli roasted turkey
- ½ (8 ounce) package reduced-fat cream cheese, softened
- 2 teaspoons chopped fresh dill weed or 1/2 teaspoon dried dill weed
- 1 medium carrot, coarsely shredded
- ½ cup coarsely shredded zucchini
- ½ cup finely chopped red sweet pepper

Instructions

- On each slice of turkey, spread cream cheese. Sprinkle with dill weed. Top with carrot, zucchini and sweet pepper. Tightly roll up turkey slices. Cover and chill for 1 hour or until ready to serve. Cut rolls crosswise into 1-inch slices.

Nutrition Info

51 calories; total fat 3g 5%, saturated fat 2g; cholesterol 15mg 5%, sodium 154mg 6%, potassium -1mg; carbohydrates 2g

61 HAWAIIAN-STYLE PUDDING

Prep Time: 5 mins
Total Time: 10 mins
Servings: 6

Ingredients

- ☐ 6 sugar-free vanilla pudding snack cups
- ☐ 1/4 teaspoon orange or almond extract
- ☐ 1 (11-ounce) can mandarin oranges, drained
- ☐ 2 tablespoons chopped roasted macadamia nuts

Instructions

- ☐ Empty pudding cups into medium bowl. Stir in extract and fold in mandarin oranges.
- ☐ Spoon 1/2 cup pudding into 6 dessert dishes and garnish with macadamias.

Nutrition Info

Calories 100
Calories from Fat 19
Total Fat 2.1g 3 %
Saturated Fat 1.3g 7 %
Trans Fat 0.0g 0 %
Protein 1.6g 3 %

62 COTTAGE CHEESE FLUFF

Prep: 5 Mins
Additional: 30 Mins
Total Time: 35 mins
Servings: 6

Ingredient

- 3 cups low-fat cottage cheese
- 2 (0.3 ounce) packages sugar-free lemon flavored Jell-O® mix
- 1 (8 ounce) container lite frozen whipped topping, thawed

Instructions

- Place the cottage cheese in a food processor and blend until creamy. Whisk in the flavored gelatin powder, then fold in the thawed whipped topping. Refrigerate until serving.

Nutrition Info

183.4 calories; protein 15.8g 32%, carbohydrates 18.2g

63 SUGAR-FREE OLD-FASHIONED BERRY COBBLER

Preparation: 15 mins
Cooking: 25 mins
Total Time: 40 mins
Serves: 8 people

Ingredients

For Berry Filling:

- 3 tbsp cornstarch
- 3 tbsp water
- ½ cup fruit-sweet boysenberry syrup or blueberry syrup
- ¾ tsp cinnamon
- 4 cups blackberries or marionberries, boysenberries, blueberries
- 1 packet sweetener up to 2 pkt, as sweet as 2 tsp sugar each, optional

For Cobbler Dough:

- 1 cup unbleached flour
- 1 ½ tsp baking powder
- ½ tsp salt
- 2 tbsp butter melted
- 2 tbsp apple juice concentrate
- ¼ cup low-fat fruit-sweet berry yogurt or cherry flavor

Instructions

- Preheat the oven to 400 degrees F. Spray a deep-dish pie pan with nonstick spray.

- Stir cornstarch into water until dissolved.

- Mix in syrup and cinnamon. Fold rinsed, drained berries into filling mixture. Let sit and set aside.

- Sift together flour, baking powder, and salt.

- In a separate bowl, combine butter, juice concentrate, and yogurt.

- Pour wet ingredients over the dry ingredients. Blend gently with a fork for 20 to 30 seconds.

- Knead the dough for 20 to 30 more seconds. On a floured surface, press dough into approximately ¼ to ½ inch thickness and wide enough to cover your pan.

- Pour berry filling into a greased pan.

- Set the cobbler dough over the top, making the dough surface as even as possible.

- Press the dough against the sides of the pan and cut a design in the dough for air vents.

- Turn the oven down to 375 degrees F and bake for 20 to 25 minutes, until the dough is light brown.

☐ Let cool and serve. Since blackberries vary in sweetness, you can sprinkle up to 2 packets of sweetener over the top if desired.

Nutrition Info

Calcium: 90mg
Calories: 132kcal
Carbohydrates: 23g
Cholesterol: 1mg
Fat: 4g
Fiber: 4g
Iron: 1mg
Potassium: 150mg
Protein: 3g

64 DARK CHOCOLATE FROZEN BANANA BITES

Active Time 12 Mins
Total Time 2 Hours 12 Mins
Servings : 18 bites (serving size: 3 bites)

Ingredients

- 3 small (about 6-in.-long) ripe bananas, each cut into 6 (1-in.) slices 18 cocktail picks 5 ounces dark (85% cacao) chocolate, finely chopped 2 teaspoons coconut oil 2 tablespoons unsweetened shredded dried coconut, toasted 2 tablespoons chopped toasted almonds 1/2 teaspoon sea salt flakes (such as Maldon)

Instructions

- Skewer each banana slice with 1 cocktail pick and place on a parchment-lined baking sheet. Freeze for 1 hour.
- Pour water to a depth of 1 inch into bottom of a double boiler set over medium heat; bring to a light boil. Reduce heat to medium-low and simmer. Place chocolate and oil in top of double boiler and cook, stirring often, until chocolate melts and mixture is smooth, about 4 minutes.
- Dip 1 skewered banana slice in chocolate mixture; immediately sprinkle with a pinch of coconut and return to baking sheet. Repeat procedure with remaining coconut for 5 more banana slices, then with almonds for 6 banana slices, then with sea salt for remaining 6 banana slices. Freeze bites for 1 hour before serving.

65 COOKIES 'N' CREAM CRUNCH

9 servings (serving size: 1 square)

Ingredients

- 1 (6 1/2-ounce) package sugar-free chocolate sandwich cookies, crushed
- 1/3 cup chopped pecans
- 3 tablespoons reduced-calorie margarine, melted
- 1 quart vanilla no-sugar-added, fat-free ice cream, softened

Instructions

- Combine first 3 ingredients; reserve 1 cup mixture. Press remaining crumb mixture firmly in bottom of a 9-inch square pan. Freeze 10 minutes.
- Spread ice cream over crumb mixture in pan. Sprinkle reserved crumb mixture over ice cream; gently press mixture into ice cream. Cover and freeze at least 8 hours.
- To serve, let stand at room temperature 5 minutes; cut into 9 squares.

Nutrition Info

232 calories; calories from fat%; fat 10.1g; saturated fat 1.7g; mono fatg; poly fatg; protein 6.3g; carbohydrates 34.2g; fiber 0.7g

66 SUGAR FREE LEMON PIE - LOW CARB + GRAIN FREE

Prep Time: 20 mins
Cook Time: 20 mins
Total Time: 40 mins
8 people

Ingredients

- 1 Coconut flour pie crust - recipe from my blog, click link

Sugar free Lemon curd

- 1/2 cup Lemon Juice or juice of about 5 small lemons
- 2 Egg
- 2 Egg Yolk - keep egg white for meringue
- 1/2 cup Butter or coconut oil, melted
- 1/4 cup Erythritol -erythritol or monk fruit sugar

Soft sugar free meringue frosting

- 2 Egg White
- 1/4 cup Erythritol

Instructions

Coconut Flour Pie Crust

- Prepare the
- Coconut flour Pie Crust

Sugar Free Lemon Curd

- Whisk the lemon juice, sweetener, eggs and egg yolks together in a sauce pan.
- Bring to medium heat and add the coconut oil or butter, stirring continuously, to prevent the eggs from cooking and scramble.
- When the coconut oil is melted, increase the heat to medium-high, keep stirring until it thickens up.
- When thick, remove from heat and transfer into a bowl to cool down at room temperature for 15 minutes.
- Fill in the coconut flour pie crust with the lemon curd. Refrigerate the lemon pie for at least 2 hours to firm up.

Sugar free meringue frosting

- Before serving add the meringue.
- In a bowl whisk the egg white until it starts producing a good volume. Usually 30 seconds on high speed.
- Keep whisking on high speed and slowly add the sugar free crystal sweetener of your choice.
- After 1 minute and 30 seconds the meringue should be really fluffy and triple its volume.
- Upside down the bowl to check if the meringue is ready. If it stick to the bowl transfer on the top of the lemon curd pie.
- Torch the top of the meringue or place 2 minutes in the oven on grill more until the top is slightly brown.

67 BUNYAN'S DIABETIC SOUR CREAM BANANA CAKE

Serves: 8 to 12
Prep: 20 Min
Cook: 45 Min

Ingredients

- 1/2 stick butter, room temperature
- 1/3 c splenda's splenda sugar blend
- 2 large eggs
- 1 tsp vanilla extract
- 2 c flour
- 1 tsp baking powder
- 1 tsp baking soda
- 1 c sour cream
- 3 bananas, mashed

Instructions

- Pre heat oven to 350
- Cream butter with Splenda, sugar blend
- Add eggs & vanilla, beat well
- Sift together flour, baking powder, baking soda, & sea salt
- Add to creamed mixture alternately with sour cream
- Fold in the mashed bananas
- Spray a 13X9 baking pan with Pam
- Pour the batter into the pan
- Bake at 350 40 to 45 minutes or until done

Prep time 10 min
Servings 6

Ingredients

- 1/4 cup pecans (chopped)
- 12 cake pop sticks
- 1/2 cup blueberry Greek yogurt (non-fat)
- 12 strawberries (hulled)
- 1 Wax paper

Instructions

- Line a small baking sheet with wax paper. Set aside.
- Insert the cake pop sticks into the top part of the strawberry. Do not pierce through the end of the strawberry.
- Dip each strawberry in the yogurt, shaking so that each strawberry is thinly coated. Use a spoon to help coat the strawberries if needed.
- Sprinkle 1 Tsp. of pecans over each coated strawberry.
- Place the strawberry pops on the baking sheet and freeze for 1-2 hours or until the yogurt is frozen. Once the pops are frozen, remove from the wax paper and serve or put in a freezer zip top bag.

Nutrition Info

Calories 55
Total Fat 3.5g

Saturated Fat 0g
Cholesterol 0mg
Sodium 5mg
Total Carbohydrate 5g
Dietary Fiber 1g

69 APPLE COFFEE CAKE

Prep/Cook Time: 1 hour 20 minutes, Servings : 20 servings

Ingredients

- 5 C   tart apples, cored, peeled, chopped
- 1 C sugar or replace with 1/4 Tsp Stevia Concentrated Powder plus unsweetened applesauce
- 1 C   dark raisins
- 1/2 C pecans, chopped
- 1/4 C vegetable oil
- 2 tsp vanilla
- 1 egg, beaten
- 2-1/2 C
- sifted all-purpose flour
- 1-1/2 tsp baking soda
- 2 tsp
- ground cinnamon

Instructions

- Preheat oven to 350¼ F.
- Lightly oil a 13x9x2-inch pan.

- In a large mixing bowl, combine apples with sugar or Stevia powder and applesauce, raisins, and pecans; mix well. Let stand 30 minutes.
- Stir in oil, vanilla, and egg.
- Sift together flour, soda, and cinnamon;
- Stir into apple mixture about 1/3 at a time just enough to moisten dry ingredients.
- Turn batter into pan.
- Bake 35 to 40 minutes.
- Cool cake slightly before serving.

Nutrition Info

Calories: 188
Total fat: 5 g
Saturated fat: less than 1 g
Cholesterol: 11 mg
Sodium: 68 mg

70 BUCKWHEAT GINGERBREAD MUFFINS

Total Time 40 Mins
Servings 12 muffins (serving size: 1 muffin)

Ingredients

- 3/4 cup plus 2 tbsp. (110 g) brown rice flour
- 1 teaspoon baking soda
- 1/4 teaspoon xanthan gum*
- 1/2 teaspoon cinnamon
- 1/2 teaspoon ground ginger
- 1/4 teaspoon ground allspice
- 1/4 teaspoon salt 1 1 1/2 by 1 1/2 in. piece fresh ginger (about 40 g)
- 2/3 cup (140 g) packed light brown sugar
- 1/2 cup (1 stick; 115 g) unsalted butter
- 1/3 cup (120 g) light unsulfured molasses
- 1 large egg
- 3/4 cup plus 2 tbsp. (110 g) buckwheat flour

Instructions

- Position a rack in lower third of oven and preheat to 375°. Line 12 muffin cups with paper liners.
- In a large bowl, whisk brown rice flour, baking soda, xanthan gum, cinnamon, ground ginger, allspice, and salt together until well blended. Set aside.
- Peel fresh ginger. "I like to use a spoon because it gets around the curves better than a peeler. I peel toward me for the most control." Slice ginger very thinly across the

grain until you have 1/4 cup (30 g). Put ginger slices and brown sugar in a food processor and pulse into a purée.

- ☐ Cut butter into cubes and melt it in microwave. "Cubing it helps the butter melt evenly and helps keep it from spitting as it heats." Add hot butter, flour mixture, molasses, and egg to food processor with ginger-sugar purée and whirl 20 seconds. "Process any longer, and the xanthan gum could lose its thickening power." Scrape bowl, add buckwheat flour and 1/2 cup hot water, then process exactly 5 seconds more.

- ☐ Pour batter into a liquid measuring cup, then divide it among lined muffin cups, wiping your finger across the rim of the measuring cup to cut off the flow of batter without dripping all over the pan. The cups should be 3/4 full, using every bit of batter.

- ☐ Bake until a toothpick inserted in the center of a muffin comes out with a few dry crumbs, 15 to 20 minutes. Set muffins on a rack for a few minutes to firm up, then carefully remove from pan (tilting it helps) and set on rack to cool completely.

- ☐ Make ahead: Up to 4 days at room temperature in an airtight container; up to 3 months, frozen airtight. Bring to room temperature before serving.

71 BAKED CINNAMON STUFFED APPLES

Prep time 10 min
Cook time 30 min
Servings 8 Servings

Ingredients

- 4 large McIntosh or Golden Delicious Apples (cored)
- 1/2 lemon (juiced)
- 6 tbsp Splenda® Brown Sugar Blend
- 1/4 cup oatmeal
- 1 tsp ground cinnamon
- 2 tbsp margarine (trans-fat-free)
- 1/4 cup pecans (finely chopped)

Instructions

- Preheat oven to 425 degrees.
- Drizzle lemon juice over apples.
- In a small bowl, mix together remaining ingredients. Stuff each apple with approximately 1/4 cup oat mixture.
- Place apples in an oven safe baking dish and bake for 25-30 minutes.

72 GRILL PEACHES

Servings 6 to 8
Prep time 5 minutes
Cook time 8 minutes to 10 minutes

Ingredients

- 6 peaches, preferably freestone
- Olive oil

Instructions

- Prepare the grill. Light a gas grill to medium heat. If you're cooking over charcoal, grill the peaches after everything else has been grilled.

- Halve and pit the peaches. Run a sharp knife along each peach's seam to halve them. Remove the pit and brush each cut side with olive oil.

- Grill cut-side down, over medium heat, for 4 to 5 minutes. Place the peaches cut-side down on the grill and cook undisturbed until grill marks appear, 4 to 5 minutes.

- Flip the peaches and cook until tender, 4 to 5 minutes. Flip the peaches and grill until the skins are charred and the peaches are soft, 4 to 5 minutes more.

- Serve the peaches. Remove from the grill. Serve the grilled peaches with vanilla or butter pecan ice cream, or even as an accompaniment to grilled pork

73 SUMMER FRUIT SALAD

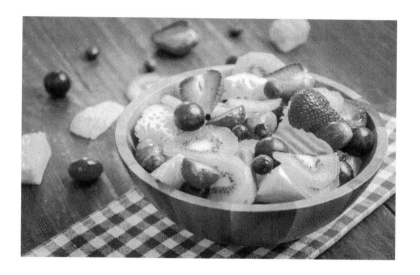

Preparation time: 30 minutes (includes standing time)
4 servings

Ingredients

- 1/2 cup fresh blueberries
- 1/2 cup fresh blackberries
- 1/2 cup fresh raspberries
- 1/2 cup fresh strawberries, hulled and sliced
- 2 medium-size ripe peaches, thinly sliced
- 1 cup seedless grapes
- 2 tablespoons fresh lime juice
- 2 tablespoons granulated sugar
- 3 medium fruit, without skins kiwi fruit, peeled and sliced

Instructions

☐ Combine the fruit in a large bowl. Combine the lime juice and sugar. Add to the fruit mixture and toss to blend. Allow the fruit salad to stand for 20 minutes before serving to allow flavors to blend.

Nutrition Info

Calories: 106 calories, Carbohydrates: 27 g, Protein: 1 g, Fat: <1 g, Saturated Fat: <1 g, Sodium: 4 mg, Fiber: 4 g

74 FIVE-INGREDIENT CHOCOLATE CHIP COOKIES

Prep: 10 Mins
Total Time: 25 mins
Servings : 30

Ingredients

- 1 cup almond butter
- 1 cup semisweet chocolate chips
- 1/2 cup packed light-brown sugar
- 2 large eggs
- 1/2 teaspoon coarse salt

Instructions

- Preheat oven to 350 degrees. In a bowl, stir together almond butter, chocolate chips, sugar, eggs, and salt until a dough forms.
- Place 1-tablespoon mounds of dough 1 inch apart on parchment-lined baking sheets. Bake cookies until puffed and tops are set, about 10 minutes.
- Transfer to a wire rack; let cool. Cookies can be stored in an airtight container up to 3 days.

75 PUMPKIN-MAPLE CRUSTLESS CHEESECAKE

Servings: 12

Ingredients

- 3 (8 ounce) packages fat-free cream cheese, warmed in a microwave for 15 seconds
- 1/3 cup Splenda Brown Sugar Blend
- 3 large eggs
- 1 (15 ounce) can pumpkin puree
- 1/2 cup low-fat maple or vanilla yogurt
- 2 tablespoons all-purpose flour
- 1-1/2 teaspoons ground cinnamon
- 1 teaspoon ground ginger
- 1 teaspoon imitation maple or rum flavoring
- 1 teaspoon vanilla extract
- 1/4 cup thinly sliced crystallized ginger (garnish)

Instructions

- Preheat oven to 350 degrees F. Coat the bottom and sides of a 9-inch spring form pan with non-stick cooking spray.
- Using an electric mixer, beat cream cheese and Splenda Brown Sugar Blend until smooth. Beat in eggs one at a time. Blend in pumpkin, yogurt, flour, cinnamon, ground ginger, maple flavoring, and vanilla.
- Pour filling into prepared pan. Bake until outer rim is puffy and center is slightly wobbly, about 1 hour and 10 minutes. Remove from oven and run a butter knife around the inner edge but do not remove the pan side. Let stand at room temperature 30 minutes. Refrigerate

warm cake, uncovered, until cold. Then cover with foil and refrigerate at least 4 hours (or up to 3 days). Remove 1 hour before serving.

- ☐ When ready to serve, carefully remove side of pan. Cut into 12 wedges with wet knife wiped clean between cuts. Garnish with crystallized ginger, if desired.

Nutrition Info

Calories: 130
Fat: 2.5 grams
Saturated Fat: 1 grams
Fiber: 1 grams
Sodium: 420 milligrams

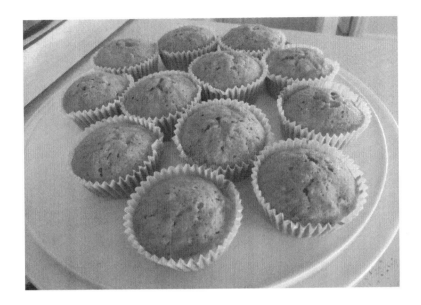

Makes 24

Cook Time 18 Min

Ingredients

- 1/2 cup canola oil
- 2 egg whites
- 1 egg
- 2/3 cup sugar
- 1 cup molasses
- 1 cup unsweetened applesauce
- 1 1/2 cup all-purpose flour
- 1 cup whole wheat flour
- 2 1/2 teaspoons baking soda
- 1 teaspoon ground ginger

- 1 teaspoon ground allspice
- 1 teaspoon ground cinnamon
- 1/2 teaspoon salt
- 1 1/3 cup reduced-fat frozen whipped topping, thawed

Instructions

- Preheat oven to 350 degrees F. Line muffin tins with paper liners.
- In a large bowl, beat the oil, egg whites, egg, and sugar until well blended. Add molasses and applesauce; mix well.
- In a small bowl, combine the flours, baking soda, ginger, allspice, cinnamon, and salt; gradually beat into applesauce mixture until blended. Spoon mixture into muffin tins, filling each about 2/3 full.
- Bake 18 to 22 minutes or until a toothpick inserted near the center comes out clean. Cool completely. Just before serving, top each cupcake with 1 tablespoon whipped topping.

77 FRESH FRUIT WITH APPLESAUCE-SWEETENED TAHINI

Servings: 4

Ingredients

- 1/4 cup tahini
- 1/2 cup unsweetened applesauce
- 1 tablespoon honey
- 2 tablespoons water
- 4 cups sliced fruit, such as mango, black grapes, plums, and citrus
- 1/4 cup toasted, unsweetened coconut flakes

Instructions

- Combine tahini, applesauce,honey, and water in a foodprocessor. Pulse until smooth.Arrange fruit in serving bowls.Drizzle with tahini sauce andtop with toasted coconut.

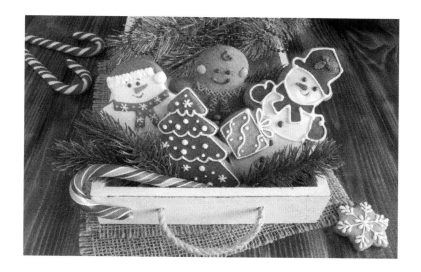

Servings: 24 servings

Ingredients

- 1/2 cup shortening
- 3 tablespoons Equal ® sugar substitute
- 1 egg
- Several drops of food coloring (optional)
- 2 1/2 cups cake flour
- 1/2 teaspoon salt
- 2 teaspoons baking powder
- 1/2 cup skim milk
- 2 tablespoons water
- 1 teaspoon vanilla extract

Instructions

- ☐ Cream shortening. Add sweetener, egg, and food coloring (if desired); beat well.
- ☐ In a separate bowl, combine dry ingredients, add the milk, vanilla, and water. Put in flour mixture and stir well.
- ☐ Chill dough 2 to 4 hours.
- ☐ Preheat oven to 325 degrees F.
- ☐ Roll out 1/8 inch thick and cut the cookies into desired shapes. Bake for 8 to 10 minutes.
- ☐ Cool. Store in air tight container.

Nutrition Info

Calories: 104
Fat: 4.5 grams
Sodium: 95 milligrams
Cholesterol: 9 milligrams
Protein: 3 grams
Carbohydrates: 12 grams

79 BANANA CHIA PUDDING

Prep: 10 Mins
Additional: 2 Hrs
Total Time: 2 hrs 10 mins
Servings: 6

Ingredients

- 1 ½ cups vanilla-flavored flax milk
- 1 large banana, cut in chunks
- 7 tablespoons chia seeds
- 3 tablespoons honey
- 1 teaspoon vanilla extract
- ⅛ teaspoon sea salt

Instructions

- Put milk, banana, chia seeds, honey, vanilla extract, and sea salt in respective order in the blender; blend until smooth. Pour mixture into a bowl and refrigerate until thickened, at least 2 hours. Spoon mixture into small bowls to serve.

Nutrition Info

112 calories; protein 1.6g 3%, carbohydrates 20.5g 7%, fat 3.4g 5%, cholesterolmg; sodium 59mg

80 ALMOND BUTTER-QUINOA BLONDIES

Total Time: 1 hr 35 mins
Servings: 24

Ingredient

- ¼ cup unsalted butter, softened
- ¾ cup smooth or crunchy natural almond butter
- 2 large eggs
- ¾ cup packed light brown sugar
- 1 teaspoon vanilla extract
- ¾ cup quinoa flour
- 1 teaspoon baking powder
- ¼ teaspoon salt
- 1 cup semisweet chocolate chips

Instructions

- Preheat oven to 350 degrees F. Line an 8-inch-square baking pan with parchment paper (or foil), allowing it to slightly overhang opposite ends. Coat with cooking spray.
- Beat butter and almond butter in a mixing bowl with an electric mixer until creamy. Beat in eggs, brown sugar and vanilla. Whisk quinoa flour, baking powder and salt in a small bowl. Mix the flour mixture into the wet ingredients until just combined. Stir in chocolate chips. Spread the batter evenly into the prepared pan.
- Bake until a toothpick inserted into the center comes out with just a few moist crumbs on it, 25 to 35 minutes. Do not overbake. Let cool in the pan for 45 minutes. Using the parchment (or foil), lift the whole panful out and

transfer to a cutting board. Cut into 24 squares. Let cool completely before storing.

Nutrition Info

147 calories; total fat 9.1g 14%, saturated fat 3.1g; cholesterol 21mg 7%, sodium 73mg 3%, potassium 101mg 3%, carbohydrates 15.5g

81 SUGAR-FREE PINEAPPLE LUSH CAKE

Prep Time: 15
Cook Time: 30
Total Time: 45 minutes

Ingredients

- 1 Pillsbury Sugar-Free Yellow Cake, prepared according to package Instructions in a 9×13 pan
- (you'll need eggs, oil, and water for the cake mix!)
- 1 (8 oz) container of Sugar-Free Cool Whip
- 1 (20 oz) can of crushed pineapple in juice (undrained)
- 1 (1.5 oz) box of Jell-O Sugar-free Instant Vanilla pudding mix (just the mix, do not make the pudding!)

Instructions

- Bake the cake in a 9×13" cake pan according to package Instructions. Allow it to cool completely!!

- ☐ In a mixing bowl, stir together the dry pudding mix, Cool Whip, and pineapple. Mix it until it's thoroughly combined!
- ☐ Spread over the chilled cake (right in the pan!) and let it to chill for at least an hour! Enjoy!!

82 MACERATED STRAWBERRIES

Prep Time 35 mins
Total Time 35 mins
Servings: cups

Ingredients

- ☐ 1 pint 1 pound, 2 cups fresh strawberries
- ☐ 2 tablespoons sugar

Macerated Strawberries with Grand Marnier

- ☐ reduce sugar to 1 tablespoon
- ☐ 2 tablespoons Grand Marnier

Macerated Strawberries with Citrus Juice

- ☐ reduce sugar to 1 tablespoon
- ☐ 2 tablespoons lemon or orange juice

Macerated Strawberries with Balsamic Vinegar

- ⬜ reduce sugar to 1 tablespoons
- ⬜ 2 teaspoons balsamic vinegar

Instructions

- ⬜ Wash, hull, and slice strawberries and place into a large glass bowl. Stir in sugar and allow to stand for 30 minutes for strawberries to release their natural juices, but not so long that they begin to become mush.
- ⬜ If using Grand Marnier, citrus juice or balsamic vinegar, add at the same time as sugar.

83 CARROT CAKE TOWERS: DIABETIC FRIENDLY

Servings: 16
Calories: 208

Ingredients

- ⬜ 1 1/2 cups all-purpose flour
- ⬜ 2/3 cup flax seed meal
- ⬜ 2 teaspoons baking powder
- ⬜ 1 teaspoon pumpkin pie spice
- ⬜ 1/2 teaspoon baking soda
- ⬜ 1/4 teaspoon salt
- ⬜ 3 cups finely* shredded carrot about 6 medium (3 large for me)
- ⬜ 1 cup refrigerated or frozen egg product thawed, or 4 eggs, lightly beaten

- 1/2 cup granulated sugar or sugar substitute blend** equivalent to 1/2 cup granulated sugar
- 1/2 cup packed brown sugar or brown sugar substitute blend** equivalent to 1/2 cup brown sugar
- 1/2 cup canola oil
- 1 recipe Fluffy Cream Cheese Frosting
- Coarsely shredded carrot optional

Instructions

- Preheat oven to 350°F. Grease the bottom of a 15x10x1-inch baking pan; line bottom of pan with waxed paper. Grease and lightly flour the waxed paper and the sides of the pan. Set aside.
- In a large bowl, stir together flour, flax seed meal, baking powder, pumpkin pie spice, baking soda, and salt; set aside.
- In another large bowl, combine finely shredded carrot, eggs, granulated sugar, brown sugar, and oil.
- Add egg mixture all at once to flour mixture. Stir until combined.
- Spoon batter into prepared pan, spreading evenly.
- Bake for 25 to 30 minutes or until a toothpick inserted near center comes out clean. Cool cake in pan on a wire rack for 10 minutes. Invert cake onto a wire rack. Cool completely.
- Transfer cake to a large cutting board. Using a 2-inch round cutter, make cutouts in the cake, leaving as little space as possible between cutouts.
- You should get 28 to 32 cutouts.
- For each serving, place one of the cake cutouts on a serving plate. Spread or pipe about 1 tablespoon Fluffy Cream Cheese Frosting atop the cake round. Top with a

second cake round and about 1 tablespoon additional frosting. If desired, garnish with coarsely shredded carrot.

Nutrition Info

Calories: 208cal, Carbohydrates: 25g, Protein: 4g, Fat: 10g, Saturated Fat: 1g, Sodium: 117mg, Potassium: 194mg, Fiber: 3g, Sugar: 12g

84 CINNAMON-BANANA CAKE WITH CHOCOLATE GANACHE

Prep Time: 15 mins
Total Time: 1 hr 15 mins
Servings: 16

Ingredients

Cinnamon-Banana Cake

- ☐ 2 cups all-purpose flour
- ☐ ½ cup whole-wheat pastry flour
- ☐ ½ cup granulated sugar
- ☐ ½ cup packed brown sugar
- ☐ 1 ¼ teaspoons baking powder
- ☐ 1 teaspoon ground cinnamon
- ☐ ½ teaspoon salt
- ☐ ½ teaspoon baking soda
- ☐ ¾ cup fat-free milk

- ½ cup refrigerated or frozen egg product, thawed, or 2 eggs, lightly beaten
- ⅔ cup mashed banana
- ¼ cup canola oil
- 1 teaspoon vanilla

Chocolate Ganache

- 3 ounces dark chocolate, chopped
- ¼ cup fat-free half-and-half

Instructions

- Preheat oven to 325 degrees F. Generously grease and flour a 10-inch fluted tube pan; set pan aside.
- To prepare Cinnamon-Banana Cake: In large mixing bowl stir together flours, granulated and brown sugar , baking powder, cinnamon, salt and baking soda.
- In medium bowl combine milk, eggs, banana, oil and vanilla. Add egg mixture all at once to flour mixture. Beat with an electric mixer on medium to high speed for 2 minutes. Spoon batter into prepared pan; spread evenly.
- Bake about 45 to 55 minutes or until a wooden toothpick inserted near the center comes out clean. Cool in pan on a wire rack for 10 minutes. Remove cake from pan. Cool completely on a wire rack.
- To prepare Chocolate Ganache: In a small microwave-safe bowl combine chocolate and half-and-half. Microwave, uncovered, on 50% power (medium) for 1 minute. Let stand for 5 minutes. Stir until completely smooth. Let stand to thicken slightly.
- Spoon evenly atop cooled cake.

Nutrition Info

197 calories; total fat 5.4g 8%, saturated fat 1.3g; cholesterol 1mg; sodium 177mg 7%, potassium 121mg 3%, carbohydrates 33.8g

85 MINI ECLAIR BITES

Chill Time 4 Hr
Cook Time 5 Min
Servings S 18

Ingredients

- 2 cups reduced-fat graham cracker crumbs
- 1/2 cup confectioners' sugar
- 1 1/2 stick margarine, melted
- 1 (4-serving size) package sugar-free instant French vanilla pudding mix
- 1 1/4 cup lowfat milk
- 2 cups fat-free frozen whipped topping, thawed
- 3/4 cup sugar-free chocolate frosting

Instructions

- Preheat oven to 350 degrees F. Line 18 mini-muffin cups with paper liners.
- In a medium bowl, combine graham cracker crumbs, sugar, and butter; mix well. Evenly press mixture into paper liners. Using your fingers, press over bottom and up sides of liners.
- Bake 5 minutes, or until crust begins to brown. Remove from oven and cool completely.
- In a medium bowl, whisk pudding mix and milk. Fold in whipped topping. Place in a resealable plastic bag and snip off one corner. Fill graham cracker crusts evenly with pudding mixture.

In a small microwave-safe bowl, heat frosting 10 to 15 seconds; stir until smooth and pourable. Place in a small resealable plastic bag and snip off one corner. Top pudding mixture with a dollop of chocolate frosting. Refrigerate 4 hours or until ready to serve.

Nutrition Info

Calories 178
Calories from Fat 93
Total Fat 10g 16 %
Saturated Fat 2.0g 10 %
Trans Fat 2.1g 0 %
Protein 1.1g

86 SUGAR-FREE APPLE PIE

Prep/Cook Time: 1 hour, Servings: 4

Ingredients

- 12 oz. unsweetened apple juice concentrate, thawed
- 3 Tbsp. cornstarch
- 1 Tbsp. ground cinnamon
- 6 cups tart apples, thinly sliced
- 2 9-inch pie shell pastries

Instructions

- Preheat the oven to 350 degrees. In a small bowl, whisk together 1/3 cup of the apple juice concentrate with the cornstarch and cinnamon.
- Set aside. In a large saucepan, combine apples and remaining apple concentrate.
- Bring to a simmer over medium heat and cook until the apples are tender, around 10 minutes.
- Stir in the cornstarch mixture and cook for an additional five minutes.
- Remove from heat. Place one of the pastries into your pie dish, then spoon in the apple mixture. Roll out the remaining pastry so it fits over the top of the pie. Gently place it over the filling, then seal and flute the edges.
- Cut a few steam vents in the top of the crust.
- Bake the pie for 45 minutes or until the crust is golden brown.

87 DIABETIC CHOCOLATE NUT COOKIES

Prep/Cook Time: 30 min, Servings: 4

Ingredients

- ▯ 1 sq. unsweetened chocolate
- ▯ 1/3 c. butter
- ▯ 2 tbsp. li▯uid sweetener
- ▯ 2 tsp. vanilla
- ▯ 2 eggs, beaten
- ▯ 1 c. sifted cake flour
- ▯ 1/2 tsp. salt
- ▯ 1/2 tsp. baking soda
- ▯ 3/4 c. chopped walnuts

Instructions

- ▯ Melt unsweetened chocolate and butter in saucepan over low heat. Add li▯uid sweetener, vanilla and beaten eggs. Stir until well blended. Stir in chopped walnuts. Pour into a greased 8x8 pan. Level in pan. Bake in slow oven at 325 for 20 minutes. Cool and cut into bars. Makes 32 cookie bars, each contains 55 calories. 2 bars = 1 1/4 bread exchange and 2 fat exchange.

88 FRUIT COMPOTE A LA MODE

Prep Time: 15 mins
Total Time: 1 hr 15 mins
Servings: 8

Ingredients

- 1 1/4 cups water
- 1/2 cup unsweetened orange juice
- 1 12-ounce package mixed dried fruit (dice larger pieces of fruit)
- 1 teaspoon ground cinnamon
- 1/4 teaspoon ground nutmeg
- 1/4 teaspoon ground ginger
- 4 cups fat-free vanilla frozen yogurt

Instructions

- Combine water, orange juice, dried fruit, cinnamon, nutmeg and ginger in a saucepan and place over medium heat. Gently stir and simmer for 10 minutes, covered.

- Remove the cover and continue to simmer over very low heat for an additional 10 minutes or until the fruit is soft.

- Serve warm or cold in bowls with vanilla frozen yogurt.

Nutrition Info
Total carbohydrate 47 g
Dietary fiber 5 g
Sodium 68 mg

Cholesterol 3 mg
Protein 5 g

89 SUGARLESS SPICE CAKE

This scrumptious cake is bursting with the flavors of autumn. It's sure to be a hit with everyone at your holiday gathering, and they won't even realize it's made for diabetics!

Ingredients

- 2 cups raisins
- 2 cups water
- 1 cup unsweetened applesauce
- 2 eggs, beaten
- 2 Tbsp. liquid artificial sweetener
- 3/4 cup vegetable oil
- 1 tsp. baking soda
- 2 cups all-purpose flour
- 1 1/2 tsp. ground cinnamon
- 1/2 tsp. ground nutmeg
- 1 tsp. vanilla extract

Instructions

- Preheat your oven to 350 degrees and coat an 8-inch square baking dish with cooking spray. In a small saucepan, combine raisins and water.
- Cook over medium heat until the water has evaporated.
- Remove from heat and add in the applesauce, eggs, sweetener and oil.

▢   Stir well to combine. Use a whisk to blend in the baking soda and flour. Finally, stir in the remaining ingredients, then pour the mixture into the prepared baking dish. Bake for 25 minutes or until a toothpick inserted into the middle of the cake comes out clean. Cut the cake into small squares to serve, and garnish with a dollop of sugar-free whipped topping if you desire.

90 PEANUT BUTTER SWIRL CHOCOLATE BROWNIES

Prep Time: 15 mins
Total Time: 40 mins
Servings: 20

Ingredients

- ☐ Nonstick cooking spray
- ☐ ¼ cup butter
- ☐ ¾ cup granulated sugar
- ☐ ⅓ cup cold water
- ☐ ¾ cup refrigerated or frozen egg product, thawed, or 3 eggs, lightly beaten
- ☐ ¼ cup canola oil
- ☐ 1 teaspoon vanilla
- ☐ 1 ¼ cups whole-wheat pastry flour, divided
- ☐ 1 teaspoon baking powder
- ☐ ¼ cup creamy peanut butter
- ☐ ½ cup unsweetened cocoa powder
- ☐ ¼ cup miniature semisweet chocolate pieces

Instructions

- ☐ Preheat oven to 350 degrees Fahrenheit. Line a 9x9x2-inch baking pan with foil, extending foil up over the edges of the pan. Lightly coat foil with nonstick spray. Set aside.
- ☐ In a medium saucepan, melt butter over low heat; remove from heat. Whisk in sugar and the water. Whisk in egg, oil and vanilla until combined. Stir in 1 cup of the flour and the baking powder until combined (batter will be thin at

this point.) Place peanut butter in a small bowl; gradually whisk in 1/2 cup of the batter until smooth. Set aside. In another bowl, combine the remaining 1/4 cup flour and the cocoa powder. Stir into the plain batter; stir in chocolate pieces. Pour chocolate batter into prepared pan.

▢ Drop peanut butter batter in small mounds over chocolate batter in pan. Using a thin metal spatula, swirl batters together. Bake for 20 to 25 minutes or until top springs back when lightly touched and a toothpick inserted near the center comes out clean. Cool completely in pan on a wire rack. Cut into bars.

Nutrition Info

151 calories; total fat 8g 12%, saturated fat 3g; cholesterol 6mg 2%, sodium 61mg 2%, potassium -1mg; carbohydrates 17g

91 SUGAR-FREE GERMAN CHOCOLATE CAKE

Prep/Cook Time: 40 minutes

Ingredients

Cake

- 3/4 cup unsweetened cocoa powder
- 1 1/2 sticks melted butter – divided (1 stick softened, 1/2 stick melted)
- 1 cup unflavored Greek yogurt
- 3/4 cup Truvia baking blend
- 4 eggs separated
- 2 whole eggs
- 2 tsp vanilla
- 2 1/4 cup all purpose flour
- 1 tsp baking soda
- 1/2 tsp salt
- 1-2 cups buttermilk

Pecan Frosting

- 12 oz can evaporated milk
- 1/3 cup Truvia baking blend
- 1 egg
- 1 Tbsp all purpose flour
- 2 Tbsp butter – cut in small pieces
- 2 tsp vanilla
- 1 1/2 cup unsweetened coconut
- 1/2 cup chopped pecans

Instructions

CAKE

- ☐ Preheat oven to 350 degrees
- ☐ Spray 3-8 or 9 inch round baking pans with non stick spray and line the bottoms with parchment paper
- ☐ Sift flour, soda and salt together and set aside
- ☐ In large bowl, beat 4 egg whites until stiff peaks form, set aside
- ☐ In a medium bowl, mix 4 Tbsp (1/2 stick) melted butter with cocoa powder then add Greek yogurt to form a paste – set aside
- ☐ *I recommend using a hand mixer for this. I stirred by hand and it left some large clumps of cocoa powder. I think using the mixer would help incorporate everything better*
- ☐ In a large bowl of stand mixer, cream 8 Tbsp (1 stick) butter with Truvia until fluffy
- ☐ Add the 4 egg yolks, one at a time, beating after each addition
- ☐ Add the 2 whole eggs, beating again
- ☐ Now, add the vanilla and chocolate paste blending until well combined
- ☐ Alternate adding flour mixture and 1 cup buttermilk
- ☐ If the batter is thicker than normal cake batter add up to 1 extra cup of buttermilk until the proper consistency has been achieved. DO NOT add more than 1 extra cup or the cake will not set properly
- ☐ Remove bowl from stand and gently fold in beaten egg whites
- ☐ Bake at 350 for 20-25 minutes or until toothpick inserted into center comes out clean

- When cakes are done, turn the oven off, crack the door and leave them in 5 minutes before removing to baking rack to finish cooling
- When pans are cool enough to handle, remove cakes and allow to cool completely before frosting

FROSTING

- In a small sauce pan combine all ingredients except vanilla and nuts
- Cook, stirring freuently, on medium-low heat until thick
- Remove from heat and stir in vanilla and pecans
- Allow to cool a couple of minutes before frosting
- Place first layer on cake stand or plate
- Spread about 1/3 of frosting on cake and place another layer on top. Repeat with remaining 2 layers
- Sides of cake can be left un-frosted or covered with canned sugar-free chocolate frosting
-

92 LOW CARB BOUNTY BARS

Prep Time: 10 mins
Total Time: 30 mins
20 bars

Ingredients

- 2 cups unsweetened desiccated coconut
- 1/2 cup Canned Coconut cream shake the can before use, full-fat minimum 30% fat, at room temperature (not cold)
- 1/3 cup Erythritol
- 1/3 cup Coconut oil , melted, at room temperature

Chocolate coating

- 6 oz Sugar-free Chocolate Chips
- 2 teaspoon Coconut oil
- 1-2 Monk Fruit Drops or Stevia Drops - optional, adjust to taste

Instructions

- Cover a square pan 9 inches x 9 inches with parchment paper. Set aside
- In a food processor, add melted coconut oil, desiccated coconut, erythritol and canned coconut cream (shake can before use!).
- Process for at least 1 minute on high-speed. You may have to process 20 seconds, stop, scrape down the bowl and repeat until it comes together into a fine wet coconut batter.
- Press the raw dough onto the prepared pan, making sure there is no air left between the batter. I like to press the batter with my hands first and then flatten the surface with a spatula.
- Freeze 10 minutes to firm up. Don't freeze them too long or they get super hard and it is difficult to cut them into bars, and they break in pieces easily, still delicious but less pretty as it's more difficult to shape bars.
- Remove from the freezer, lift up the parchment paper to release the coconut block from the pan easily and place on a chopping board.
- Use a sharp knife (warm blade under a flame to avoid the bars to break in pieces!). Cut into 20 rectangles.

- ⬚ If you want, shape each rectangle into your hands to form round borders like the real bounty bars.
- ⬚ Place each formed bounty bars on plate covered with parchment paper and set aside in the freezer while you prepare the chocolate coating.
- ⬚ Meanwhile, melt the sugar free chocolate chips with coconut oil in the microwave. Microwave by 30 seconds bursts until fully melted. Add stevia drops to adjust sweetness to your taste if desired.
- ⬚ Using two forks, dip each coconut bars into the melted chocolate mixture. Return each dipped bars onto the plate covered with parchment paper or on a cooling rack. When all the bars has been covered with chocolate, freeze again 10 - 15 minutes to set the chocolate shell.
- ⬚ Store the bounty bars in an airtight container in the fridge for up to 4 weeks or freeze. Defrost 30 minutes before eating.

Nutrition Info

Calories 169.7 Calories from Fat 122
Fat 13.6g21%
Fiber 5.6g23%
Sugar 0.8g1%
Protein 0.7g

93 DARK CHOCOLATE ALMOND BARK WITH SEA SALT

Prep Time 5 mins
Cook Time 15 mins
Total Time 20 mins
Servings 10 pieces

Ingredients

- 50 g cocoa butter about 1/2 cup
- 1/2 cup unsweetened cocoa I used Ghirardelli
- 1/4 cup low carb sugar substitute or 1 tbsp+ 2 tsp Truvia
- 1/8 teaspoon sea salt
- 1/2 teaspoon vanilla extract
- 1/4 cup almonds chopped
- 1/8 teaspoon sea salt optional
- 1/4 teaspoon almonds finely chopped, optional

Instructions

- Melt cocoa butter in a chocolate melter or double boiler.
- Stir in cocoa powder, sweetener, and salt.
- Keep on heat until dry ingredients have been well incorporated into the melted cocoa butter.
- Remove from heat. Stir in vanilla extract and chopped almonds.
- Pour out on prepared pan or chocolate mold.
- Sprinkle with additional salt and chopped almonds if desired.

Nutrition Info

139 calories, 14g fat, 64mg sodium, 5.7g carb, 0.5g fiber, 4.8g erythritol, 0.4g net carb, 2.6g protein

94 COCONUT FRUIT S'MORES

Prep: 25 Mins
Broil: 3 Mins To 4 Mins
Servings: 12

Ingredient

- 4 ounces dark or semisweet chocolate, chopped
- 3 tablespoons butter, melted and cooled
- ⅓ cup flaked coconut
- 12 marshmallows
- 1 ⅓ cups fresh blackberries
- 24 graham cracker squares

Instructions

- Preheat broiler. Place chocolate in a small microwave-safe bowl. Microcook on 50 percent power (medium) for 1-1/2 minutes. Let stand for 5 minutes. Stir until smooth. Let cool for 10 minutes.
- Place butter and coconut each in a shallow dish; roll marshmallows in butter and then coconut. Thread berries and marshmallows on 6-inch skewers and place on prepared baking sheet. Sprinkle any remaining coconut atop marshmallows. Spoon chocolate onto half of the graham crackers and arrange on a platter.

- ⬚ Broil skewers 3 to 4 inches from heat for 1 to 1-1/2 minutes or until coconut is lightly browned and marshmallows are puffed, turning once halfway through broiling.
- ⬚ To serve, immediately top each chocolate-coated graham cracker with a skewer. Use remaining graham cracker to pull marshmallows and berries off skewers and form sandwiches. Makes 12 servings.

Nutrition Info

150 calories; total fat 9g; saturated fat 5g; polyunsaturated fat 1g; monounsaturated fat 3g; cholesterol 8mg; sodium 120mg; potassium 107mg

95 SUGAR-FREE GUMMY WORMS

Serves 7 (makes 28)
Prep 5 min
Chill time 2 hr

Ingredients

- 2 packages (4-serving size) sugar-free gelatin (any flavor)
- 2 (0.13-ounce) envelopes unsweetened soft drink mix* (like Kool-Aid, any flavor)
- 3/4 ounce (3 envelopes from a 1 ounce box) unflavored gelatin
- 1 cup boiling water

Instructions

- Coat an 8-inch square baking dish with cooking spray.*

- In a medium bowl, combine all the ingredients until dissolved. Pour into the baking dish, cover, and chill for 2 to 3 hours, or until completely set.

- Cut into 1/4-inch strips to form thin "worms" for serving as is or decorating other treats.

Nutrition Info
Calories 14
Calories from Fat 0
Total Fat 0.0g 0 %
Saturated Fat 0.0g 0 %
Trans Fat 0.0g 0 %   Protein 3.7g

96 DIABETIC ALMOND MACAROONS

Prep Time: 20 minutes
Cook: 60 minutes
Serving 4 dozen

Ingredients

- 1 each egg white
- 1/4 cup sugar or (replace sugar with 1/16 Tsp Stevia plus 1/3 cup unsweetened applesauce)
- 1 teaspoon almond extract
- 1/4 cup wheat germ

Instructions

- Preheat oven to 325 degrees F.
- In a deep bowl, beat egg whites on low speed of an electric mixer until frothy.
- Beat on high speed until stiff.
- Gradually beat in sugar (or Stevia) and then almond extract.
- Fold in wheat germ (and applesauce.)
- Drop mixture by 1/2 teaspoonsful onto a cookie sheet that had been sprayed with
- a nonstick cooking spray and dusted lightly with flour.
- Put the cookies in the oven and immediately reduce the temperature to 200
- degrees F
- Bake 1 hour.
- Turn off heat, and leave cookies in oven to cool.

Nutrition Info

Calories 74
Total Fat 1.0g 1%
Saturated Fat 0.0g 1%
Trans Fat 0.0g
Cholesterol 0mg 0%
Sodium 1mg 0%

97 CHEWY "TURTLES" COOKIES

Prep Time: 20 minutes
Cook Time: 15 minutes
Cooling time (caramel): 2 hours
Servings: 18 cookies

Ingredients

Cookie Dough

Dry Ingredients

- 3/4 cup almond flour
- 2 tbsp coconut flour
- 2 tbsp tapioca flour
- 1/2 cup organic cacao powder
- 3/4 tsp Himalayan salt

Wet Ingredients

- 1/2 cup ghee
- 1/2 cup raw honey
- 1 large egg
- 1 tbsp full fat coconut milk
- 1 tsp pure vanilla extract (or make your own

Chewy Caramel

Part I

- 1 cup coconut sugar
- 1/4 cup water

Part II

- 1/2 cup full fat coconut milk
- 1/2 cup coconut sugar
- 1/4 cup raw honey
- 3 tbsp ghee, or make your own
- 1 vanilla bean, seeds scraped
- 1 tsp Himalayan salt

Garnish

- Chewy caramel, you'll need about 3/4 of the above recipe
- 1/4 cup raw pecans, chopped
- 18 pecan halves
- 50 g dark chocolate, melted

Instructions

- In a medium mixing bowl, whisk the flours, tapioca starch, cacao powder and salt together, then sift. For best results, I strongly recommend that you do not skip this step. It's the best way to ensure that all the lumps get broken down (coconut flour is especially lumpy) and any potential larger pieces or unwanted debris get caught.

- ☐ Add ghee and honey to a separate bowl and beat on high speed with an electric mixer until smooth and creamy. Add egg, coconut milk and vanilla extract, cream some more until light and fluffy.

- ☐ Add dry ingredients and mix on low speed until barely just combined, no more. Finish mixing the batter by hand with a rubber spatula or wooden spoon. Transfer the cookie batter to the refrigerator, uncovered, and let it cool for at least 2 hours.

- ☐ Meanwhile, start working on the chewy caramel: in a medium saucepan, mix the coconut sugar and water listed under "Part I" and bring to a boil over medium-high heat. Let the mixture boil for about 3 minutes, until it takes a really dark caramel color and starts getting thicker.

- ☐ Meanwhile, in a separate saucepan set over medium heat, mix all the ingredients listed under "Part II" and cook, stirring occasionally, until the mixture just barely starts to simmer then kill the heat. It is important that you do not let this come to a full boil.

- ☐ As soon as Part I is ready, slowly pour in the warm coconut milk mixture while constantly stirring with a wooden spoon.

- ☐ Once all the milk has been added and completely incorporated, bring the caramel to a boil and continue cooking for 3 full minutes while stirring constantly, then turn off the heat, transfer to a small bowl and set aside to cool.

- When the caramel is cool enough and has the consistency of soft toffee, preheat your oven to 350°F and line a baking sheet with parchment paper.
- Roll the dough into 1" balls (roughly the size of a ping-pong ball) and place them at least 1" apart on the baking sheet. A spring loaded ice cream scoop works wonders for this!
- Sprinkle each cookie with chopped pecans then make an indentation in their center by pressing down gently with your finger.
- Bake the cookies for 8 minutes and remove from oven. Immediately press centers again to recreate the indent. Cool for 5 minutes in the baking sheet and then transfer to a wire rack.
- With wet hands, grab about a teaspoon of caramel from the bowl and shape it into some kind of a flat circle. Place that flat circles right into the cookies' indents. Don't worry about shaping the centers perfectly; the warmth of the cookies will take care of that for you in just a few minutes. If you find that your caramel is too stiff and won't flatten nicely, place it in the microwave for just a few seconds (really, a FEW, as in 5 to 10) to make it a tad more pliable, or place the cookies in the warm oven for a minute or two after having placed the caramel centers on all of them.
- Lightly press half a pecan over each of the caramel centers and then drizzle with the melted dark chocolate.
- Place the cookies in the refrigerator to cool completely and then store in a single layer in a cool, dry place for up to a week.

Nutrition Info

Calories: 209kcal, Carbohydrates: 27g, Protein: 2g, Fat: 12g, Saturated Fat: 7g, Cholesterol: 28mg, Sodium: 260mg, Potassium: 61mg, Fiber: 2g

98 DIABETIC-FRIENDLY PERFECTLY POACHED PEARS

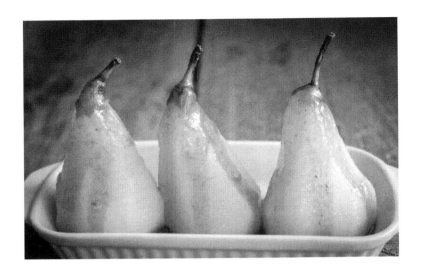

Serves: 4
Prep: 10 Min
Cook: 30 Min

Ingredients

- 1 c orange juice
- 1/4 c apple juice
- 1 tsp ground cinnamon
- 1 tsp ground nutmeg
- 4 whole pears
- 1/2 c fresh raspberries
- 2 Tbsp orange zest

Instructions

- In a small bowl, mix together orange juice, apple juice, ground cinnamon and nutmeg.
- Stir ingredients until evenly mixed and set aside.
- Peel pears, leaving the stems.
- Remove the core from the bottom of the pear.
- Place pears in a shallow sauce pan.
- Pour juice mixture over pears into pan and set over medium-heat.
- Simmer pears for 30 minutes, turning frequently.
- DO NOT BRING LIQUID TO A BOIL!
- Transfer pears to individual serving plates.
- Garnish plates with raspberries and orange zest.
- Serve immediately and enjoy!

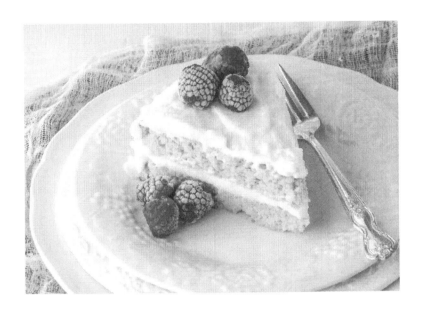

Prep Time: 45 mins
Total Time: 1 hr 20 mins
Servings: 16

Ingredients

Vanilla Cake

- ¾ cup fat-free milk
- ¼ cup butter
- ½ vanilla bean
- 3 eggs
- 1 ¼ cups sugar
- 1 ½ cups all-purpose flour

- ☐ 1 ½ teaspoons baking powder
- ☐ ¼ teaspoon salt
- ☐ 1 ½ teaspoons vanilla extract

Coconut Cream Frosting

- ☐ 4 ounces reduced-fat cream cheese
- ☐ 2 tablespoons unsweetened refrigerated coconut milk
- ☐ ¼ teaspoon coconut extract (optional)
- ☐ 1 cup frozen light whipped dessert topping, thawed

Honey & Fruit Topping

- ☐ 1 tablespoon honey
- ☐ ⅛ teaspoon ground ginger
- ☐ Pinch ground cardamom
- ☐ 1 cup assorted fresh fruit (such as raspberries, halved strawberries, coarsely chopped mango, coarsely chopped pineapple, and/or sliced kiwifruit)
- ☐ 2 tablespoons large flaked unsweetened coconut, lightly toasted

Instructions

- ☐ In a small saucepan combine 3/4 cup fat-free milk and 1/4 cup butter. Using a small sharp knife, split 1/2 of a vanilla bean lengthwise in half. Scrape the seeds from the halves into the milk mixture. Add the vanilla bean halves to the saucepan. Heat over medium heat until butter is melted and milk is steaming, stirring occasionally (do not boil). Remove from the heat.
- ☐ Preheat oven to 350 degrees F. Meanwhile, grease and lightly flour two 8-inch round cake pans. In a large bowl

beat 3 eggs, room temperature, with a mixer on high about 4 minutes or until thickened and light yellow in color. Gradually add 1 1/4 cups sugar , beating on medium speed 4 to 5 minutes or until light and fluffy. Add 1 1/2 cups all-purpose flour, 1 1/2 teaspoons baking powder and 1/4 teaspoon salt. Beat on low to medium just until combined.

- Remove the vanilla bean halves from the milk mixture; discard. Add milk mixture to batter along with 1 1/2 teaspoons vanilla, beating until combined. Divide batter between prepared pans, spreading evenly. Bake about 25 minutes or until a toothpick inserted near centers comes out clean. Cool cake layers in pans for 10 minutes. Remove layers from pans; cool on wire racks.
- In a bowl beat 4 ounces reduced-fat cream cheese (Neufchâtel), softened, with a mixer on medium until smooth. Gradually beat in 2 tablespoons unsweetened refrigerated coconut milk until smooth. If desired, beat in 1/4 teaspoon coconut extract. Fold in 1 cup frozen light whipped dessert topping, thawed.
- In a bowl stir together honey, ginger and cardamom.
- To assemble, place one cake layer on a cake platter. Spread with half of the Coconut Cream Frosting. Repeat layers. Toss fruit with honey mixture and arrange on cake. Sprinkle with coconut. Serve immediately.

Nutrition Info

189 calories; total fat 6.4g 10%, saturated fat 3.9g; cholesterol 48mg 16%, sodium 148mg 6%, potassium 76mg

100 DIED AND WENT TO HEAVEN CHOCOLATE CAKE,DIABETIC VERSION

Ready in: 1hr
Serves: 10

Ingredients

- 1 3/4 cups all-purpose flour
- 1/2 cup Splenda granular
- 1/2 cup Splenda brown sugar blend
- 3/4 cup cocoa powder
- 1 1/2 teaspoons baking powder
- 1 1/2 teaspoons baking soda
- 1/2 teaspoon salt
- 1 1/4 cups low-fat buttermilk
- 1/4 cup vegetable oil
- 1/2 cup Egg Beaters egg substitute
- 2 teaspoons vanilla extract
- 1 cup hot strong black coffee

Instructions

- Preheat oven to 350 degrees F.
- Grease a deep cake pan or bundt with non-stick cooking spray, set aside.
- Blend flour, SPLENDA Granulated Sweetener, SPLENDA Brown Sugar Blend, baking powder, baking soda, cocoa powder and salt in large mixing bowl.
- Combine buttermilk, oil, EggBeaters, vanilla extract, and coffee in a small bowl.

- Add flour to mixture, using an electric mixer on medium speed, mix until Smooth (about 2 minutes).
- Pour batter into cake pan or bundt pan.
- Bake for 35 minutes, until an inserted toothpick in center of cake comes out clean. Let cool in pan for 5 minutes.

101 CHOCOLATE MOUSSE

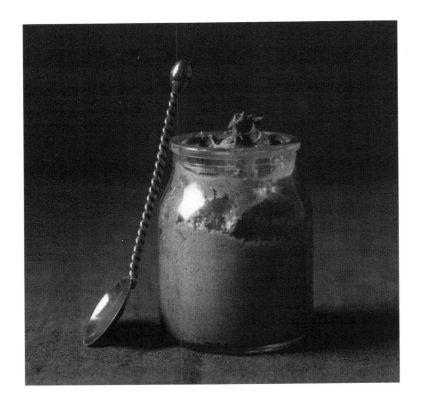

Servings: 6
Prep Time: 25 minutes

Cook time: 5 minutes
Total Time: 30 minutes

Ingredients

- 7 oz (2 bars) Perugina or Ghirardelli bittersweet or dark chocolate
- 2 Tbs strong coffee (I use decaffeinated espresso)
- 2 Tbs orange liquor OR Bourbon (optional)
- 2 medium egg yolks
- ¼ cup granulated sugar substitute
- 1 tsp pure vanilla extract
- ¾ Cup + 3 Tbs whipping cream
- 3 medium egg whites

Instructions

- Break up 5 ounces of the chocolate. Place the chocolate, coffee, and liquor In a small pot. Cover and place the small pot in a larger pot of hot water that has been turned off the heat (this prevents scorching). Allow to melt.

- Beat together egg yolks and sugar substitute until frothy. Add the 3 Tbsp. whipping cream and the vanilla to the egg mixture and beat to combine.

- Whisk the melted chocolate until smooth and shiny. SLOWLY add the melted chocolate to the egg mixture, stirring constantly.

- Beat egg whites until stiff peaks form. Fold in ¼ of the egg whites to the chocolate to lighten the mixture. Fold in remaining egg whites.

- Grate the remaining 2 ounces of chocolate on the medium side of a box grater. Fold into the mixture.

- Beat the 3/4 cup of whipping cream until tripled in bulk and holds its shape. Fold the whipped cream into the rest of the mixture.

- Pour into six individual dessert glasses or into one large bowl.

- Chill for 4-5 hours.

Nutrition Info

Calories: 168; Carbs: 7g; Fat 10g; Protein 10g; Sodium 138mg; Sugar 5g.

CONCLUSION

One of the main goals for a diabetic diet is to lower your weight and maintain it. In addition, the diet is designed to help maintain regular glucose levels in your body. Diabetes prevents your body from processing glucose the way it should, so a diabetic diet has to, to some degree, perform that maintenance. In addition, the hope is that a diabetic diet will also help you to maintain healthy lipid levels and keep your blood pressure under control.

And, a diabetic diet will vary some from person to person. The benefits and assistance to your body from the diabetic diet will depend on what type of diabetes you are trying to treat. Each type has its own challenges and level of restriction on the diet. The important thing to remember, though, is that studies show the effectiveness of a diabetic diet is dependent, not so much on the diet itself, but on how well the patient follows the diet. Given that information, there are still some specifics to keep in mind.

Made in the USA
Las Vegas, NV
02 December 2024

13237123R00103